THE DOCTORS' CASE AGAINST THE PILL

Also by Barbara Seaman

WOMEN AND THE CRISIS IN SEX HORMONES
FREE AND FEMALE

BARBARA SEAMAN

THE DOCTORS' CASE
AGAINST THE PILL

With a Foreword by
The Boston Women's Health Book Collective

A Dolphin Book
Doubleday & Company, Inc., Garden City, New York
1980

Library of Congress Cataloging in Publication Data

Seaman, Barbara.
  The doctors' case against the pill.

  (A Dolphin book)
  Includes bibliographical references and index.
  1. Oral contraceptives—Side effects. I. Title.
[DNLM: 1. Contraceptives, Oral—Popular works.
QV177 S439d]
RG137.5.S37   1980   613.9'432

Copyright © 1969, 1980 by Barbara Seaman
ISBN: 0-385-14575-6
Library of Congress Catalog Card Number 78-8202
Dolphin Books
Doubleday & Company, Inc.
All Rights Reserved
Printed in the United States of America

This book is for my daughters, Elana and Shira—
and for my son, Noah

FOREWORD

The Pill was and is the first mass chemical contraceptive in the history of the world, which over 90 million women worldwide still take. It was launched with government approval as a gigantic experiment without adequate study and testing, but most women, and even most physicians, did not know this at the time. They did not know that the early testing involved only 132 women in Puerto Rico, that there were several deaths resulting from the Pill, and that many women dropped out of the testing. Very few women were followed up. Even more alarming, as early as 1962 G. D. Searle & Co., a major manufacturer of the Pill, had records of more than one hundred reports of thrombosis and embolism, including 11 deaths.

Ten years ago, in 1970, the questions raised in the first edition of this book were being debated at Senator Gaylord Nelson's hearings on the Pill. The purpose of those hearings was not, as many people supposed, to determine its safety. Already on the market since 1960, the Pill had been approved by the Food and Drug Administration as "safe." Rather, the issues at the hearing were informed consent and the patient's right to complete information. Fortunately, because of Barbara Seaman's efforts and the spontaneous participation of other women concerned about the risks of the Pill, the safety question *was* raised at these hearings.

This book, the Nelson hearings, and the continuing work of many health feminists were responsible for the eventual mandate requiring patient package inserts (PPI's) for birth control pills. The PPI established a major historical precedent in relations among the drug industry, the Food and Drug Administration, the medical profession, and the consuming public. For the first time our government conceded that women (patients) should not be required to depend on their physicians for adequate information about the risks and benefits of a drug. Instead, manufacturers were required by the government to supply certain information directly to the "patient."

More recently, this important right to informed consent was upheld once again when the Pharmaceutical Manufacturers Association (PMA) and the American College of Obstetricians and Gynecologists (ACOG) failed in their efforts to block the requirement of PPI's in estrogen replacement therapy products (1977–78). Thanks to the efforts of the FDA and four consumer groups, including the National Women's Health Network, this PPI now warns women that they have a demonstrated seven to fifteen times greater risk of developing endometrial cancer after exposure to menopausal estrogens than women who do not take them.

The new material assembled in this book brings the present evidence against the Pill to alarming proportions. As authors of *Our Bodies, Ourselves,* we get hundreds of letters each year from women in our country and from other countries telling us their experiences with drugs and contraceptives developed by U.S. manufacturers. We feel it is crucial that their reports be acknowledged and validated, and that they be given full information about the risks they are taking. We wish women all over the world would read this book, as it probably would convince many of them not to take the often unforeseeable risks that have already produced so much regret on the part of so many women.

Even though its sales are dropping in the United States, the Pill is still on the market and at least 40 million prescriptions are filled each year worldwide. This raises many questions for

us about the direction of new contraception in the future.
What kind of protection will governments provide to the
women and children of the world against dangerous drugs and
devices of the future? How will we protect ourselves from the
unpredictable, long-term damaging health consequences? We
know that U.S. drug manufacturers have influenced what kinds
of birth control will be available to women in other countries
through repeated bribes of bureaucrats in foreign governments.
We also know that a policy of population control that makes
individual women expendable is now gaining popularity around
the world.

As you read the new and complete story of the Pill, these are
the issues we hope you will keep in mind. As you understand
how many, how crippling, and how unpredictable the Pill's side
effects are, we hope you will think whenever possible of how to
protect yourself, or a daughter, or a friend. Just as important,
we hope you will help to change our government's policies, so
that stories like the Pill (and DES and Depo-Provera) won't
continue to happen and won't happen again to unsuspecting
women and children somewhere else in the world.

Judy Norsigian
Norma Swenson
The Boston Women's Health Book Collective
February 1980

INTRODUCTION

According to the Western medical model, pregnancy is a disease, menopause is a disease, and even not being pregnant is a disease. Dangerous drugs and devices are given to women, but not to men—just for birth control. After more than twenty years of medical reporting, I've reached the conclusion that to many doctors *being a woman is a disease*.

I reject that notion. I think that being a woman is perfectly normal for . . . about half the population. Unfortunately, the half for whom it is normal don't supply us with enough doctors or medical researchers. Consider China, where more than a third of the doctors and scientists are female. In China, they have a Pill for men.

In most Western countries, the doctors are men and the patients are women. Men don't even enter the health care system until they reach middle age. They don't go for regular checkups until a friend drops dead playing tennis or jogging.

Consider how, by contrast, a woman is made dependent upon her doctor through so many of the key episodes of her life, episodes that are critical to her self-definition, her self-respect, her very identity.

A young girl gets her first menstrual period and sometime thereafter, as part of this process of becoming a woman, she gets her first pelvic exam. The doctor will charge twenty-five, fifty dollars or more and he won't even bother to warm up the speculum. If the young girl is a DES daughter—and there are 3 or 4 million of them just in the United States—the first exam is terrifying beyond description. It may be painful as well. And bear in mind that DES abnormalities are entirely iatrogenic, or doctor-created. Because the girl's mother was given an unproved, ineffective, totally unnecessary hormone, the girl must live with the fear of cancer and infertility.

Next our young woman falls in love. Back she may go to her doctor for contraception. For economic reasons, doctors like to control contraception. They downgrade the drugstore methods, the "greasy kid stuff," and many teenagers don't even know that condoms and foam are highly reliable when they are carefully used.

Nor do most doctors like bothering with the diaphragm or cervical cap, or teaching how to do ovulation timing (rhythm) properly. A doctor's time is money, and he knows it. It takes an hour or more to help a beginner select the right barrier method and coach her until she is confident. In contrast, it takes but a few minutes to insert an IUD, or write a Pill prescription and push it across a desk. The Pill has over one hundred proven side effects, so only a doctor with a very slow practice would bother to discuss them all. However, a few family planning centers and clinics are very well staffed with trained and sympathetic birth control counselors or other health workers, often volunteers, who do take great pains to discuss the advantages and drawbacks of each method and help every client make a selection that is suitable for her.

If she does not find a satisfactory birth control method, the young woman soon returns to her doctor for an abortion. About 1 million teenage women become pregnant every year, and one in three decide to terminate.

An early abortion need not be painful, but most doctors and commercial clinics are in too much of a rush to use local anesthesia with care. A surgeon can do up to four abortions an hour if he does not fuss with pain-killers. He can do only two or three if he is more solicitous. Abortionists sometimes admit to deliberate sadism. The head of a large clinic in New York City once told me, "We don't fuss too much with anesthesia because we don't want those girls coming back in here every six months."

In time our young woman will probably want to have a baby. Many doctors act as if the baby is *theirs*. How often I've heard obstetricians running through the halls of hospitals calling out, "We're in labor."

It's true that there are some women who have the philosophy "Knock me out, Doctor, and wake me when the hairdresser shows." But other women may not want to subject their babies to drugs or anesthesia. They and their husbands, or other friends and relatives, may want to participate in the birth. Surely this should be the patient's choice and not the doctor's.

The right to natural childbirth was won by laywomen who fought for it strenuously in this country for many years. Doctors succumbed to it, with resentment, only when the evidence that labor-inducing drugs and anesthesia could harm the baby had mounted very high.

But now the doctors have a new toy, fetal monitors, and they are using it as promiscuously as little boys do pop guns. Natural childbirth in the hospital is gravely threatened, and the Cesarean section rate is climbing to scandalous proportions. Midwives who are doing home births (and have an excellent safety record) are being attacked by physicians' organizations and, in some areas, are at risk of being put out of business.

Cesarean sections are dangerous, and they are expensive, but they're faster than a normal labor, so they save the doctor time. The argument used for them is that they are "rescuing" more high-risk babies. No doubt more babies are being saved, but more mothers are lost.

Our typical patient reaches her thirties and is finished with childbearing. Her doctor is apt to ask her if she wants to be sterilized. He calls the operation "Band-Aid" surgery and makes it sound safe and simple. He doesn't tell her that there is a good chance she'll have worsened menstrual cramps, or that she might die or have serious complications at the time of the surgery. He doesn't tell her that her tubes could grow back together, as part of a long-term healing process, and produce an ectopic pregnancy up to twelve years later. Sometimes he does not even tell her that the operation is permanent, or that the male vasectomy is cheaper and safer.

Should she start having "woman's troubles," he may try to talk her into hysterectomy, removal of her womb. Close to half of the hysterectomies performed in the United States are unnecessary, and that's why Blue Cross is urging its subscribers in many areas to get a free second opinion.

Menopause . . . Estrogen products such as Premarin, which is derived from pregnant mares' urine and which (since farmers are practically willing to give this away) are extremely high-profit items, have been proved to cause not only cancer, but gallbladder disease, high blood pressure, and a host of other serious complaints.

Estrogens do curb hot flashes but are not remotely a "youth pill" or antidepressant, as manufacturers and doctors try to claim. Until the FDA clamped down, in the mid-1970s, half of the menopausal women in this country were taking estrogens for an average of ten years or longer. Most of them did not need it, for no more than 10 or 15 percent of women have troubling hot flashes. Most women sail through their menopause, without paying it much attention. Even the hot flashes are not a dangerous complaint. They reflect a period of adjustment when reproduction is gearing down, just as the high-to-low voice register changes in some adolescent males reflect a period of adjustment when reproduction is gearing up.

Menopause, in the negative, frightening sense of the word, has been in large measure a doctor-created complaint. Many women are starting to teach each other how to get through it with pride and comfort, and without drugs. Good exercise and nutrition (certain requirements do change), a positive outlook, and a wholesome life are all that is usually required.

Many gynecologists and obstetricians are excellently trained to look after emergencies and treat disease. But overall, in the care of well women, they may have done more harm than good. We must stop thinking of ourselves as "patients" when it comes to our normal processes. We must think of ourselves as people instead, people who attend to our own body signals, inform ourselves, and try to take good care of our health. In the future, it is quite possible that obstetrics-gynecology will be much smaller specialties, which, as is proper, attend to genuine ills. A different group of specialists, who are more prevention-minded, more gentle and less hurried, will be our instructors or coaches through our normal female events.

These would include nurses, midwives, nutritionists, birth control counselors, exercise instructors, and other health workers who are *not* trained to view womanhood as a disease.

I became a medical writer for personal reasons. When Noah, my son, was born in 1957, I was twenty-two years old. In the hospital I was given a packet of pills to take at four-hour intervals. I was breast-feeding, but the other three women in my ward room were not. I noticed that we were all being handed the same packets, and I wondered about that. My common sense told me that nursing mothers should probably be wary of chemicals.

I tried to find out what the pills were. The nurses and doctors wouldn't tell me. In fact, they stood over me to ensure that I swallowed my medicine.

Noah grew very sick. He developed severe diarrhea, turned yellow, and lost a lot of weight. His pediatrician—a woman and an old-fashioned naturally oriented doctor—discovered the problem. I was being given a chemical laxative that should never be prescribed to nursing mothers, for it does go into the milk.

Not long afterward, I wrote my first article: on how to subvert the breast-feeding practices in hospitals. It drew a good response, and I soon became a medical columnist or editor at several women's magazines. During the 1960s the new contraceptives—the Pill and, to a lesser extent, the IUD—were the major items of medical "news" for women. These became part of my "beat." Doctors were saying the Pill was great, but users often wrote to me with horror stories. I gave what the patients said as much weight as what the doctors stated. For example, Dr. John Rock, co-developer of the Pill, claimed that women would be "super-fertile" when they stopped. I collected hundreds of case histories from women who had the opposite experience. Their periods never came back.

Next I tried to find neutral sources: basic research scientists who had no interest in population control, in defending the Pill, or in protecting any colleagues against malpractice lawsuits. Most of the time the basic research scientists supported the women. They told me, for example, that post-Pill infertility was only to be expected. They showed me research papers, which I could hardly fathom (and I don't think that most physicians can fathom them either), explaining how hormones act like a sledgehammer on the entire reproductive system.

To prepare myself for the first edition of this book, I applied for, and received, an Advanced Science Writing Fellowship at the Columbia University School of Journalism. Some of my professors, especially John Foster, greatly bolstered my belief that I *should* believe what "ordinary" patients said. My editors, Peter and Barbara Wyden and Lois Chevalier, were also of this conviction.

The book was published in 1969. I was attacked as a yellow journalist in publications such as the New York *Times*. Christopher Lehmann-Haupt said that my book was scatterbrained and undocumented, and made him want to take the Pill by the hand and comfort it. Dr. Alan Guttmacher, director of Planned Parenthood, walked off the David Frost TV show, on which we were mutual guests, and said that he would be damned if he would "listen to all this crap." (The word *crap* was bleeped.) Margaret Mead made fun of me on the Dick Cavett program (it later turned out that she had a consultant arrangement with Planned Parenthood, which she had concealed), and I jousted with Peter Lawford on the Mike Douglas show.

But the book found support in unexpected places. The science editor of the Washington *Post*, and his equivalent at many other newspapers, treated it more than respectfully. The FDA Commissioner, Herbert Ley, praised it in public, as did HEW Secretary Robert Finch. Curiously, my reviews in scientific journals were usually more supportive and thoughtful than I would have anticipated. Senator Gaylord Nelson and Ben Gordon, his staff assistant, were sufficiently convinced to call hearings. As a result of the hearings, the patient package inserts that I had proposed were adopted by the FDA. I had never argued that the Pill should be banned (we all make some compromises with our own good health—who, for example, exercises as much as she knows she ought?), but only that users get enough information to make a free choice.

To me, the most important support for the book came from early health feminists. Alice Wolfson and her colleagues at Washington, D.C., Women's Liberation demonstrated at the Nelson hearings. They helped me clarify just how sexist an issue modern contraception really is. Later, Gloria Steinem, Nina Finkelstein, and other editors at *Ms.* magazine helped to keep the questions viable and greatly honored me by selecting this book (which had gone out of print) as one of the principal publications of the modern women's movement. Betty Friedan has always been a brilliant adviser and ally on all of the central issues in women's health. Lois Gould, who worked with me at the *Ladies' Home Journal* in the 1960s, encouraged my early skepticism about the Pill. So did her husband, Dr. Robert Gould. Barbara Youncker, the distinguished health reporter at the New York *Post*, who, among her other achievements, exposed thalidomide, was always a role model and a source of encouragement.

I am in the process of getting divorced from Gideon Seaman, M.D., my psychiatrist husband. Nonetheless, he did encourage me to follow my convictions about the Pill. So did my gynecologist, Dr. Arthur Davids, and my internist, Dr. Clifford Spingarn. Dr. Philip Corfman, chief of Contraceptive Research at the National Institute of Child Health and Human Development, and his late wife, Eunice, a Quaker of extraordinary purpose, wisdom, and humor, were unfailing sources and friends.

Finally, I want to thank Lindy Hess and Regina Ryan, the editors who so encouraged me to bring out this revision. And I am very grateful to Laura Van Wormer for her help. I want to thank Martha Aldridge and, above all, Chris O'Neil for their superb assistance with the details of the work. I want to thank my son, Noah, the circumstances of whose birth made me a health feminist. As this revision appears I am exactly twice his age—forty-four to his twenty-two—so I have known him, and been a health feminist, for exactly half my life.

I am sad, in a way, that the early Pill users I heard from or interviewed turned out to be right. I would prefer that they, and I, had been wrong, and that the Pill had proved "safe." I hope that what we have all learned from this is to trust our own experience and *not* to be intimidated by "authorities," or degrees.

Barbara Seaman
April 1980

CONTENTS

THE DOCTORS' CASE AGAINST THE PILL

CHAPTER 1

Who Takes the Pill?

The Pill is an effective contraceptive, and it counters the aesthetic or sexual objections that many couples have to barrier methods such as the diaphragm and condom. For a time it also seemed to counter the moral objections that some religions have to contraception: it was promoted by Dr. John Rock and others as "natural."

The synthetic chemicals in the Pill were given the names of female hormones, estrogen and progesterone. Many women were told, and came to believe, that all they did were mimic the natural monthly cycle.

Nonetheless, it is still hard to believe that the Pill was so widely and casually accepted. Doctors are not unintelligent. From the beginning they knew that the Pill worked by inhibiting the normal interaction of sex hormones and the pituitary gland. Because these interactions are so basic to our lives and health, the Pill was bound to have widespread serious effects.

After two decades of research, we are able to enumerate those effects: the Pill is a proven and accepted causative agent in cerebrovascular and heart diseases and causes a bizarre array of nutritional aberrations. It is strongly suspected of causing diabetes, some cancers, and arteriosclerosis.

Of the eight leading causes of death among American women, the Pill is associated with the five named above. These five cause 75 percent of the female deaths in the United States each year, and this list does not even consider the "minor" side effects of the Pill, ranging from urinary infections to sterility.

There are many reasons—in addition to a history of blood or heart disease, age, and smoking habits—why a doctor might not prescribe the Pill for a particular woman. They include histories of hepatitis, jaundice, gallbladder disease, depression, benign breast disease, migraine, fibroid tumors of the ovaries, unexplained menstrual difficulties, high blood pressure, high cholesterol, impaired glucose tolerance, or family histories of cancer or diabetes. Toxemia during a previous pregnancy or the birth of an extra-large baby are also considered contraindications by some doctors.

Nonetheless, at least 4 million women in the United States still take the Pill.

Why do doctors prescribe it?

"I think the biggest problem is a sophisticated type of ignorance," said a professor at a leading medical school. "It's not that doctors don't want to read. It's that they haven't got the time."

As well as sophisticated ignorance, there may be sophisticated laziness and greed. It takes time to fit a diaphragm or cervical cap properly, and time for the woman to learn how to insert it and check its placement. It takes a lot less time to write a prescription. The fee for both services is the same in most cases, and the Pill patient will need to return for more frequent checkups.

But why do intelligent women, aware of at least some of the dangers and complications connected with the Pill, persist in taking it? One answer is that not all of them do persist. About half the women who start on the Pill stop taking it within two years—and not because they wish to become pregnant. They stop because they are afraid of the effects they have been learning about. Or because they begin to experience intolerable discomfort, psychically or physically. Or because their doctors advise them to.

They stop because they have a friend, or a friend has a

friend, or a sister-in-law, or a neighbor who suffered a distressing reaction to the Pill. Perhaps a blood clot that left a woman with a weak and permanently swollen leg. Perhaps a reaction that caused disfiguring facial blotches. Or perhaps the Pill seemed to trigger a rapid growth of fibroid tumors so that a hysterectomy became necessary. One woman told us she stopped because of her mother-in-law's persistent nagging.

"If anything happens to you, Marjorie," her mother-in-law kept saying, "don't count on *me* to look after the children."

But what about the women who start on the Pill and have not yet stopped? Why are these presumably intelligent women still taking the Pill? There are interesting and complex reasons why women are subjecting themselves each day to unnecessary health risks.

"Infantile omnipotence, that's why," says Dr. Sandor Lorand, a psychoanalyst who began practicing medicine in Europe as a gynecologist and later became a disciple and student of Sigmund Freud.

"They think, 'It can't happen to me,'" Dr. Lorand explains. "Many immature people have this sense of immunity. They look at the world through rosy-colored glasses. Tragedy can befall other people, but not them."

This is also why many people keep smoking cigarettes and close their eyes to the well-documented dangers of lung cancer. Regardless: infantile omnipotence is for infants. When the baby is hungry, he cries. When he cries, he is fed. When he wants his mother, he cries and his mother appears. For a period during infancy, a baby naturally acquires the idea that he has magic powers. If he develops normally, this belief is outgrown, but many people retain certain aspects of it. They drive without seat belts. They smoke. They use the Pill.

"Mature people know that God has given them no special exemption," Dr. Lorand says. "Immature people, those with a sense of infantile omnipotence, do not weigh the consequences of taking the Pill. They think it's an easier way of pleasure."

A *question of motives*

There may well be a residue of infantile omnipotence in doctors who still prescribe the Pill, and in women who persist in using it. The reasons women give for using it, however, range from the ludicrous to the tragic. For instance: bigger bosoms.

One woman who went on the Pill and who lost her sex drive told us, "It's terrible. Sex used to mean a lot to me. But for the first time in my life I have a real bosom. I always felt so inferior. I used to wear falsies or at least a padded bra. And I always felt phony. Once, in the swimming pool, one of my falsies came out and just floated away. I was a laughingstock."

Another woman, twenty-six years old, happily married, with "two adorable children," said, "I suppose that once I was married, being flat-chested shouldn't have bothered me so much. It didn't bother my husband. But I always felt so cheated. I felt I had the figure of a ten-year-old boy, although my husband said it wasn't true.

"I know the Pill is dangerous," this mother told us, "but I plan to stay on it come hell or high water. And if they withdraw it, I'm going to get those silicone shots. They're dangerous, too. I know it. I don't care."

Infantile omnipotence?

Well, certainly infantile.

A study at Johns Hopkins University, involving eighty-four women seeking breast "augmentation" surgery, provides insight into the kind of woman who stays on the Pill because she is so proud of her enlarged breasts. The women in this study had a history of small breasts since adolescence. Childbearing, paradoxically, tended to give them an "increased sense of deformity." The researchers speculated that these women may have been hoping that pregnancy and birth would permanently enlarge their breasts—and then felt disappointed when their expectations failed to materialize.

The psychological profile of these women showed they were active, competitive, on the go. Most were physically graceful and attractive and appeared to be socially at ease. But underneath they showed signs of "hysterical seductiveness, depressive trends, feelings of anxiety and despair." They shared a deep thirst for recognition of their feminine attractiveness and desirability. And when this group was compared with another group of patients seeking nose surgery, it was found that many more of the breast-obsessed women had had unhappy childhoods. No wonder that such women are highly motivated in favor of the Pill.

Other women told us that they keep on taking the Pill because it does "wonders" for their complexions. A medical librarian who had tried six different oral contraceptives over a three-year period, despite constant headaches, nausea, and leg cramps that used to wake her four and five times a night, said she put up with the effects of the Pill for so long because "my complexion had never looked so beautiful. All the little pores disappeared. I hardly needed makeup."

Appearance meant a lot to this woman. "I didn't mind the nausea too much," she said, "because I was losing a lot of weight with all that throwing up." But finally even this Pill enthusiast had enough. She told us, "Eventually I got too thin and weak and I had to give the Pill up."

It may sound almost incredible that a woman—and a medical librarian at that—would go through such agony for three years for the sake of a better complexion. But our review of hundreds of case histories convinced us that she was not atypical.

One middle-aged woman told us that she is still on the Pill because she wants to fool the man she loves: "I lied to him about my age. I'm forty-eight and I've stopped menstruating, but he thinks I'm forty-two. How many women stop having periods when they're only forty-two? I think he may be a little suspicious as it is. I'm older than he is, you see."

Some women say that they know the risks of the Pill but are willing to accept them for the sake of the spontaneity it allows in their sex life. One young and extremely attractive stockbroker, married to a successful architect, explained, "I'm half kidding, but only half kidding, when I say we've decided to live by—what was it? The F. Scott Fitzgerald philosophy? Well, anyhow, *you* know: Live fast, die young, have a good-looking corpse. We have our own little plane, and sometimes, if there's a party we don't want to miss, we take it up in weather that other pilots wouldn't fly in. There are also two kinds of skiers, you know: some who only ski the trails they're sure of, and others who are always looking for a greater challenge. Well, we belong to those others. Just call us Jean-Claude Killy.

"And as far as sex goes," she continued, "well, we want to be able to do it in unexpected times and places. That's half the fun. We're finished with that greasy kid stuff forever. If my doctor forced me to give up the Pill"—she flung back her long hair emphatically—"I'd just go ahead and get my tubes tied. Or Jim would have a vasectomy [male sterilization operation]."

(Brilliant as this stockbroker may be with figures, she is not well informed about birth control. There is, for example, at least one harmless method that would give her just as much spontaneity as the Pill. The cervical cap can stay in place for days or even weeks at a time, without a change of spermicide.)

Some women take the Pill fully cognizant that they are living on borrowed time. Claudia L., a Los Angeles housewife, who had been taking the Pill for only a few months, developed suicidal impulses. She was intelligent enough to associate these with the Pill and informed her doctor immediately. The doctor put her on another brand. The switch seemed to work. Claudia is no longer suicidal. But as she herself says, "I feel as if I'm going against nature. I *know* these pills are fighting other elements in my body. I'm sure it's only a matter of time before the symptoms begin again—the same ones or other ones."

Why is Claudia, happily married and the mother of two young children, still taking the Pill? Why is she willing to risk leaving her children motherless or to condemn them to life with a mother who can become so chronically depressed because of the potency of the Pill that she may not function normally? How can she face the fact that if her symptoms recur, her marriage may break up? Or that her husband, whom she loves, may face the task of raising their two sons by himself?

"It's the safest method of contraception," Claudia explains. "The only one I trust almost 100 percent. Once my younger boy gets into kindergarten, I think I'll switch. We don't want to have a third child, but by the time Michael gets into kindergarten, I'll be able to cope with a third child if I have to.

"Also," Claudia added, "our country house will be paid off and so will our boat. Steve and I both came from families that had high standards but no money. We've always had to work hard for everything. Now we feel entitled to the pleasures of life. They are very important to us.

"But don't get me wrong"—Claudia leaned forward earnestly —"I'm not going to stay on the Pill forever. Not with two children to raise. Just three more years. I know it's too risky."

Claudia is one of the millions of women who have been convinced that the Pill is necessarily the most effective contraceptive. It is not. And as we shall discuss shortly, this misplaced trust can have heartbreaking consequences.

Another woman who still takes the Pill is Joan R., who is afraid of losing her husband. Joan is black-haired, fair-skinned, and animated. One would think she was in her twenties. Actually she is thirty-six. Her husband is exceptionally charming and witty. He is a television producer, in a treacherous job, as Joan sees it, since he is continually surrounded by aspiring young actresses. Joan and Bill have a six-year-old son and a nine-year-old daughter. Both children were planned. For the first ten years of her marriage, Joan had used a diaphragm. She hated it. She felt that it interfered with the spontaneity of lovemaking. But she did have confidence in it.

Six years ago, during Joan's second pregnancy, she began to worry about her husband's loyalty. "It's not so unusual," she maintains. "So many of my friends' husbands are leaving to marry younger women, it's getting harder and harder to get up a dinner party!" She had a difficult pregnancy and her doctor vetoed sex relations. Bill was then working with an assistant producer, a woman whom Joan describes as extremely attractive and intelligent. She is not certain that Bill had an affair with this assistant, but she is convinced that he thought about it. "I don't even have to wonder what would have happened if the sex moratorium had gone on much longer."

Joan decided, after the baby was delivered, that she had to make sex more exciting for her husband. Bill had always resented her getting up to insert the diaphragm. He used to say, "Why don't you do it automatically? When you brush your teeth, put in the diaphragm. If we don't make love that night, so what? And if we do, we don't have to be bothered." Joan had tried to follow this advice, but she found it humiliating: "After I'd gone through the whole messy business of putting it in, and he'd just turn over and go to sleep."

Joan told her gynecologist that she'd like to try the Pill. He did not want to prescribe it for her. When she told him why she wanted it, he suggested that Bill use a condom. He told her that certain higher-priced condoms made of sheep intestine interfere less with a man's sensations than the ordinary types made of rubber. Bill tried them. He found them a nuisance, grumbled a lot, and reproached Joan for being a "fraidycat" about trying the Pill. At just this time, very close friends of theirs (the woman had been one of Joan's bridesmaids) got divorced. The man had fallen in love with a younger woman. This triggered Joan's decision: "Rather than lose my husband, I was going to try the Pill—dangerous or not."

Joan has experienced very little discomfort from the Pill. Some nausea at the beginning, yes, but, she says, "it was nothing to speak of. Much less than the morning sickness I had during my pregnancies." Occasionally she has a slight watery vaginal discharge.

In spite of this good record—and Joan has maintained this arrangement for five years—her doctor is not happy. He shows her articles reporting changes in blood sugar that occur in women who take the Pill, and changes in triglyceride levels (which could indicate heart problems). At her last checkup the internist reminded Joan that her father had died of a heart attack and that her aunt had diabetes. He urged her to face the fact that the Pill was probably bringing about subtle changes in her body that might eventually shorten her life.

After the most recent checkup, Joan was almost convinced that she should stop the Pill. "Wouldn't it have been wonderful," Joan asks sadly, "if the Pill had turned out to be the miracle we all hoped it would be? I'm an adult, though, and I don't want to fool myself. In my heart I know my internist is right and that I've played around with this lovely but dangerous toy long enough. Something can happen to me, like diabetes or heart trouble, ten years from now even if I stop the Pill today."

In this country, the Pill was indeed a "lovely toy" for the middle class, peculiarly suited to their life-style. A woman who bought plastic-wrapped everything, who did not worry about the additives that let her store food for months on end, and who lived confidently with air pollution, water pollution, and nuclear reactors was not likely to worry about that tiny pill in its sterile plastic wrap.

But the times did change. Nitrites, saccharin, red food dyes, and the hair dye scandal competed for newspaper space with stories about the horrors of the Pill. Now the somewhat older, wealthier, and married Americans are dropping the Pill: they're back with the diaphragm and have access to backup abortions and eventual sterilization. Today over 20 percent of married American couples have one or more sterilized partner.

But the 4 million women who still take the Pill represent a new Pill horror: evidence that it is now a drug prescribed mainly for the very young and the very poor. Two of every three birth control patients at family planning clinics in the United States in 1977 took home a prescription for the Pill. Pill-pushing at these clinics represents a public scandal and should embarrass both the clinics and the private and public funding agencies that support them. For doctors in private practice no longer recommend the Pill to most of their patients; overall, the percentage of couples using birth control pills is now only 20 percent, despite the much larger percentage of Pill users among those who go to family planning agencies.

The very young women who need birth control represent a

peculiar set of problems for clinic personnel; they are considered "too immature" to be fitted for a diaphragm and the IUD is apt to give cramps. The rate of unwanted pregnancies among teenagers is very high: as many as one out of three sexually active teenagers will get pregnant. But the Pill is an especially poor choice for these girls. First, the long-term carcinogenicity of the Pill has not been determined, but other estrogens have been proven to cause cancer. It is suspected that the carcinogenic effects may be even more powerful in a young person. Further, the estrogens cause shortening of bones and may stunt the growth of immature women.

Many doctors refuse to prescribe the Pill for women who have never had a child. There is substantial evidence that infertility is most likely to result when the woman is quite young, has not had a child, and has an irregular menstrual cycle before beginning the Pill.

The Pill also increases a woman's chances of getting VD, which is a major public health problem among sexually active teens. And more than half of today's young women are sexually active before nineteen.

The fact that poor women and students are given the Pill while their more affluent neighbors are not indicates that we still have a two-class society as far as the practice of medicine is concerned. Doctors make a lot of assumptions about their patients: for example, in answering such questions as will she follow orders; does she understand the procedure; is she motivated enough to use another method of contraception, such as the diaphragm or the condom? How doctors answer these questions to themselves may well be affected by their personal attitudes toward women of a certain color, race, economic status, or age. Trained nurses and paraprofessionals who take time to coach women in the use of barrier or ovulation timing methods —in their own language—have been widely successful in providing contraception without medical risks.

Some doctors in the family planning movement have also come to believe that they have a greater responsibility to "society" than to individual patients.

At the 1969 meeting of the Association of American Medical Colleges, a Nobel Prize winner who had made a tremendous contribution to the health of individuals all over the world delivered a statement that left many doctors in the audience gasping. The Nobel Prize winner, Dr. Frederick C. Robbins, dean of Case Western Reserve University School of Medicine in Cleveland and one of the pioneers in the conquest of polio, told the medical educators:

"The dangers of overpopulation are so great that we may have to use certain techniques of conception control that may entail considerable risk to the individual woman."

No wonder the doctors in the audience gasped. They had been trained to think of themselves as committed to the health of each patient in their care. Suddenly they were faced with the staggering question of whether they should give priority consideration to social issues, to society at large. Suddenly each doctor seemed required to ask: "Should I take possible risks with my individual patient in order to preserve the human race, or am I committed to think first about my own patient?"

Most doctors would undoubtedly respond that their responsibility to the individual patient still comes first. But others may have come to believe that they must be social engineers as well. Their feelings toward the poor are reflected in a survey recently conducted in a midwestern city. Ninety-two percent of obstetrician-gynecologists maintained that welfare mothers should be forced to be sterilized after the birth of their second child.

Middle-class women do still take the Pill, of course, as well as opting for voluntary sterilization. There are some women who have never been successful with other methods, or who worry about pregnancy so much that they feel they need the Pill. Others seem to be caught in poor relationships with the men they love.

Winnie T. is a case in point. She is thirty-six, and just beginning to enjoy real success as a lawyer. Her lover, she told us, seems determined to get her pregnant. "He wants to make love every time I'm not prepared. When we're out, he'll suggest we stop at a hotel for the 'excitement,' instead of going back to my place. For a while I just put in the diaphragm every time I was going to see him, but he really got angry at that. He asks me not to use it if I just had my period, or other times when I'm supposed to be 'safe.' I suppose he wants to prove he's the boss, or something."

Winnie was lucky enough to find a responsible gynecologist, who reminded her about all the risks of the Pill. "Finally she handed me a form that really scared me out of taking the Pill. It listed a number of complications that women my age are likely to get. And she said that I was the one who wanted the Pill, and she was not responsible. That did it. I just told Larry we would use the diaphragm all the time, or we would break up." They are still together.

Many husbands also pressure their wives to stay on the Pill, often without being aware of it. One such husband is Evan G., whose wife, Antoinette, is the child of a former Supreme Court Justice. She grew up among special people—informed, responsible, intelligent folk who were intimately involved in some of the most significant legal and social problems of the times. Antoinette felt like a very special, privileged little girl. Her family imparted to her a heavy, if not oppressive, sense of social responsibility.

When she married Evan, he seemed like a man who "had everything." Evan was second in his class at law school. Everyone agreed that his future was not only promising, it was bound to be brilliant. He rose rapidly through the ranks of one of New York's most prestigious law firms and became a full partner before he was thirty. Antoinette pictured herself as a future Supreme Court Justice's lady.

But Evan had a weakness. Even as a law student he drank too much, although he had always seemed to be under control. By the age of thirty, however, he was undeniably an alcoholic. Because of Antoinette's contacts and those of his late father-in-law, he is still tolerated by the older partners in his firm. He does bring in business, and there are periods when he shows his former competence and promise.

Antoinette loves him and would not dream of leaving him. He is never cruel, never abusive, unfailingly charming. He is also childishly impulsive, particularly about sex. "If it happens in the middle of the day, he just drags me off into the bedroom," Antoinette says. "And I'm lucky if I can get him to do *that*. If it were up to him, he'd have me on the living-room floor, right in front of the children."

Antoinette takes the Pill, because, as she says, "I certainly can't count on Evan to use precautions. I can't even count on him to give me enough time to use a diaphragm. The IUD? I don't like them either. Besides, Evan is just the type who might pull it out for a joke. Some men do that, you know. As a social worker, I've seen it."

A study headed by a psychiatrist, Dr. Frederick Ziegler, and a psychologist, Dr. David Rodgers, of the department of psychiatry of the Cleveland (Ohio) Clinic indicates that Antoinette's predicament is shared by a certain type of woman who, knowing the dangers, persists in taking the Pill. The doctors studied thirty-nine couples *before* the wife went on the Pill, *while* the wife was on the Pill, and *after* the wife had stopped taking it. Husbands and wives were interviewed intensively—together and individually. Here is what the doctors found:

Almost every one of the wives in the study experienced side effects, most of them minor, during her first few months on the Pill.

The couples who decided to stop the Pill usually said they did so because of the discomfort of the side effects.

Among the couples whose wives suffered side effects, there was an almost equal division between those who decided to stop and those who kept on taking the Pill.

What made the difference between the couples who stopped and those who did not, keeping in mind that the discomfort of the side effects was approximately the same in both groups?

The most important factor, Drs. Ziegler and Rodgers concluded, is the balance of the husband-wife relationship: that is, who is boss? The doctors explain that in every family there are duties that are clearly those of the husband and others that unquestionably belong to the wife. And then there are "gray areas," or what they call "ambiguous responsibilities." For instance, who writes the checks for the monthly bills? This is not a clearly masculine or feminine responsibility.

Drs. Ziegler and Rodgers discovered that where the husband was the take-charge type who assumed most of the ambiguous responsibilities, the wife who suffered side effects was likely to go off the Pill. If, however, the wife dominated the gray areas, she was in the group that stayed on the Pill, regardless of side effects.

"One way of putting it," Dr. Ziegler says, "is that the father-knows-best families go off the Pill." And strong women with weaker husbands tend to stay on it. This may be one more way of asserting their authority, or it may simply be an expression of lack of trust in the husband.

Today's spoiled bachelors pressure women to take the Pill—but pressure is often required. Andrew M., a twenty-three-year-old engineer who lives in Philadelphia, is such a pressuring bachelor. He thinks the Pill is the greatest convenience since the invention of the automatic shift, and his availability seems to mean more to his girl friends than their own health or that of their yet-to-be-conceived children.

Andy is bright, although not as bright as he thinks; on the way up, but probably not going as high as he hopes. His neatly trimmed beard hides a receding chin and makes him look more dashing than when he was clean-shaven.

Andy has been reading *Playboy* since he was fifteen, but he did not start feeling like a playboy until he grew his beard and a promotion allowed him to buy a sports car. His introduction to sex had come in his senior year in high school: a quick but not disappointing episode with the "fast" girl in his neighborhood. He used a condom. At that stage of life, he says, he "always carried one" with him. In engineering school he had a couple of affairs and he used mostly condoms, "sometimes withdrawal, and sometimes nothing." But now Andy would not dream of using a condom—for either one of his "best girls."

"I made both my girls go on the Pill," he said. "Being in college and all, Sharon was scared. And Eileen was worried the Pill would make her fat. She's a dancer, and for a dancer that's bad. But I just put them on notice. No Pill—no Andy. Not quite that way, of course. I was very smooth.

"Sometimes I have one-night stands, too. I always ask them if they're on the Pill. If they say no, I say good-bye. Once a guy has had a taste of sex on the Pill, he just won't settle for anything less."

The Pill is also the easiest contraceptive for straying housewives to conceal from their husbands, and for Catholic women whose husbands are more opposed to birth control than they are.

Some ignorant or lazy doctors still press the Pill on women who should never take it. Susan D. lives in a small town in the West, where the local GP gave her a prescription when she married at eighteen. He would not even discuss alternative methods. After eight months she wrote to us to report that "I've had nothing but trouble . . . hair falling out, loss of energy, and cramping." Susan is particularly worried because "my family has a long history of ovarian cancer and for generations back the women have had complete hysterectomies by the time they were twenty-four."

Susan gave up the Pill because a TV discussion show alerted her to the link between her symptoms and the drug. But for many women her age the Pill's dangers are not well known. They are too young to remember all the stories that appeared in the late 1960s and early 1970s. Now researchers and the media don't show much interest in the Pill. One of the pioneers in Pill research, Dr. William N. Spellacy, told us that "when a medicine is new, and important, a lot of money is spent researching it. We studied the Pill, identified the dangers, and quantified them. Now we're looking at other problems."

But nobody, apparently, told Susan's doctor about the dangers. Or perhaps he assumed that she knew about them when she gave her "informed consent" for this treatment.

Renata Z. was in no position to give "informed" anything,

but she was still on the Pill. Her parents wrote us a worried letter in 1977, while Renata was a psychiatric patient at a hospital in a small southern city.

"The therapist decided she was about to commit suicide, so he went to her home and got her to go to a psychiatric hospital. She was put in the intensive-care part a couple of days later, because she was still bent on self-destruction, as they called it. The doctors still have her on the Pill, as they say 'that's what she wants' and she has a right to decide. . . ." Renata's depression, according to her doctors, is too severe to have been caused by the Pill, which she has taken for nine years, with a year and a half off to have a baby.

And yet modern research, published in England, shows that the suicide rate is tripled in Pill users. The chemicals in the Pill deplete vitamin B_6, which in turn alters brain metabolism, leading to depression. Suicidal women who take the Pill can often be cured with 40 mg daily of vitamin B_6. Most doctors, including psychiatrists, are ignorant of these facts, which may explain why suicide is claimed by some statisticians to be the leading cause of Pill-associated deaths.

Had Renata's therapist been better informed, he would have ordered blood tests to determine her vitamin B_6 levels.

Late in 1979 we interviewed medical students to learn how much they are taught today about the Pill. Sadly, we concluded that young doctors may be as ignorant as their very young patients.

Aaron K. is an energetic third-year student at a well-ranked institution in New York City. He promises to be a popular practitioner who combines a real interest in people with a love of his studies. He is heavily involved in a number of medical organizations and serves as a volunteer medic for several neighborhood groups. We asked him about the Pill's side effects.

Yes, he told us, he knew the Pill should not be used by those with fibroid breast disease. He was also aware that it could cause blood clots and strokes. But he believed that both conditions occurred only in older women who smoked, and that the dangers were "minimal" in others (see Chapters 3 and 5). He was not aware that the Pill changed carbohydrate metabolism, fat metabolism, or a number of other processes. While he did know that the Pill can cause trouble with the user's cervix, he did not relate that change to folic acid deficiency. And he had no knowledge of the Pill's effects on nutrition and very little knowledge about nutrition generally. "This is not my specialty," he told us. "Please remember that the entire obstetrical and gynecological training is two weeks, and the Pill is only a tiny part of it."

But perhaps the most disturbing aspect of this interview was that Aaron really believed that the Pill was far more effective than any other method. He was aware that his ob/gyn training was inadequate, but he apparently believed the advertisements in the medical journals.

"It's still safer than pregnancy," Aaron said, echoing what too many doctors told us.

Jerry L. is also a third-year student, in the same class as Aaron, but his career is likely to be quite different. He is fascinated by biochemistry and pharmacology and spends hours tracking down the hows and whys of drug reactions. Jerry knows a great deal about estrogen metabolism, although he has studied it in terms of its use with older men who have prostate cancers rather than as a contraceptive.

He was far more conservative than Aaron about the Pill and recognized that it would have long-term effects on fat and sugar metabolism, blood clotting, and various other bodily functions. But he, too, believed that it was far more effective than other contraceptive methods.

It may be that the medical profession relies so much on chemistry that it does not believe that simple barrier methods can do what a drug can do. Or it may be that these students, like most practicing doctors, get a great deal of their "education" from ads placed by the drug companies.

Both students made the astounding observation that "a woman who wants the Pill will just go to another doctor to get it." Apparently they have no faith in their own ability to convince a woman that the best contraceptive for her might not be the method she had in mind when she came in the door.

They could learn a great deal from Dr. Arthur Davids, a Founding Fellow of the American College of Obstetricians and Gynecologists, who has a private practice on Fifth Avenue in New York. His waiting room is filled with ordinary patients as well as quite a few celebrities. There may be a readily recognizable movie or TV star or at least a society woman whose picture has appeared in *Vogue* or *Women's Wear Daily*.

Dr. Davids does not like to prescribe the Pill, and he does so infrequently. How does he dissuade his fashionable clientele when these tend to be the very ladies who want so much to be "in" and chic and modern? The answer is that he talks to them —in detail and on their own terms. We interviewed three of his patients: a doctor's wife, an actress, and a young mother who, not recognizing the doctor's stature, selected him because he was "within walking distance" of her apartment. All three women affirmed that he discussed the Pill and its drawbacks at such length that they could not fail to be impressed.

The doctor's wife reported: "His jovial manner gradually gave way to professorial concern. He seemed quite happy to let off accumulated steam about some of his stubborn patients who refused to give up the Pill merely because of convenience." Under the influence of the doctor's obvious concern, this patient did not prove stubborn. She had come to ask for a Pill prescription but accepted a diaphragm instead.

The actress, a well-known beauty, said that Dr. Davids told her: "I'll have to give you the Pill if you insist on it. It hasn't been withdrawn. Doctors are still using it, but many of us don't like it any longer. I find the side effects grotesque and, occasionally, debilitating. Many Pill-takers become waterlogged, overweight, nauseated, and generally blowsy. Some develop eye troubles and ugly veins." By understanding her emotional needs and indirectly appealing to her vanity, Dr. Davids dissuaded this patient.

The third patient recalls that the doctor told her: "I don't see why any woman is willing to risk the Pill when a diaphragm, properly used, is so safe and easy. You're about the same age as my nurse's daughter. She was a healthy young woman, but after a few months on the Pill she developed a clot in the leg. She's fine now, but she had a bad time. On your way out, why don't you ask my nurse to tell you about it? These clotting problems are not uncommon, and we just don't know whom they'll strike. . . . You find the diaphragm distasteful? Let me show you how to use it with an inserter. Many women find that the inserter makes it more acceptable." Which proved to be the case for this woman, once she had talked with the nurse.

CHAPTER 2

Julie Is Not a Statistic

To five blue-eyed little girls she was "Mommy." To her husband she was "the heart of our home." To her older sister she was a "born mother. That was the thing God meant her for."

Whatever she was meant to be in life, Julie Macauley was not a statistic. She became a statistic only when she died at the age of twenty-nine from a pulmonary embolism and left her beloved husband, Tom, a widower and her children motherless.

Julie had been on the Pill for less than a year. Her husband is convinced that it killed her, and he is bitter against the doctors and drug manufacturers who he feels let death come so unnecessarily to his Julie.

"They say, 'Oh, it's only one in a thousand that's going to have trouble,'" he scoffed. "But this one in a thousand is my wife. She was the mother of five children. She was a real person. She was not a statistic."

Dr. Wood, a gynecologist in the large midwestern city where Julie lived, placed her on the Pill to regulate a long-standing menstrual irregularity. He testified in court that he had read drug company pamphlets and medical literature reporting more than 400 cases of clotting and 37 deaths among Pill users through 1964. Nevertheless, he had placed Mrs. Macauley on the Pill in 1965 without warning her of its possibly dangerous side effects.

The doctor said that he considered the statistical evidence of clotting to be "quite small. . . . I think the physician is supposed to exercise judgment. That's what I did. I felt I would be doing the lady a disservice to report it to her. You can scare a patient to death."

The fact is that Julie would not have been "scared to death" if the doctor had come straight out and told her the risks she was facing. She was not the type to be stampeded. Her sister Peggy described her to us as a solid, steady sort of person— "very quiet, very determined. She just went her own way."

She had been independent even when she was a baby. "She was so funny when she was little," Peggy said. "I was seven years older, so I remember her very well. I loved her dearly. She was tall for her age, but when she was three and four she always walked around with a little chair so she could get things she couldn't reach without having to ask for help.

"Julie got into everything, the way children do," Peggy recalled fondly. "And she was my father's pride and joy. He used to call her 'Shorty' because she was so tall. She had been a very wanted child.

"She was very tall and gangly by the time she reached her teens. She was really awkward then. And those long, gangly legs! They were always bent over chairs and things like that. I was married by that time and she used to come baby-sit for me. My oldest boy is nineteen now, a sophomore in college. He used to be Julie's biggest buddy. She loved all children, but she was exceptionally good to him. She used to read to him and take him to the movies. She was the best aunt a boy ever had. He found it very hard to take when she died."

When Julie outgrew the gangly stage, she turned out to be a real beauty. She was tall, slender, blond—altogether extremely attractive. Her friends told her she should be a model.

"She was a good student," her sister said, "but she didn't really like school. She had a good time, though. She had her own group of friends and they went to all the school functions together.

"She didn't date much at first, but when she got over that

gangly stage and started to blossom she dated quite a bit. She was going steady in her senior year. And then she met Tom the summer right after she graduated from high school."

Julie really meant it when she said she didn't like school. Her marks were good and she could have been accepted by most colleges, but she wasn't interested. She went to work at her hometown university as a secretary.

Rhythm didn't work

"I think my father was disappointed she didn't go on to college the way I did," Peggy said. "I had originally wanted to be a doctor. I was taking a premed course, but then I got married. I think Daddy wanted her to go ahead and get at least a couple of years of college. But she went out and got a job. Daddy said, 'You're costing me money by going to work. I'm losing you as a dependent.' He offered to send her to any college she wanted. But she just kind of smiled. She never fought or argued with him like I did. I have a redhead temper, but like I said, Julie just went her way, very determined, very quiet."

Anybody who knew Julie at all knew what was going to happen to her. She was going to get married and have a big family and live as happily ever after as real people ever do in real life.

"I met Julie when I was a sophomore," Tom Macauley told us. "We went together for two years before we got married, but I knew from the first that we were going to get married. We met at a student mixer. She was a friend of a girl who was dating a friend of mine. When we were courting, we used to talk about the children we were going to have. We decided we wanted a large family, perhaps seven or eight children."

Julie and Tom got married while Tom was still in college. Their first daughter, Anne Marie, arrived within the year. The Macauleys decided that they should wait until Tom was through college before having another child. They turned to the only form of birth control acceptable to them as Roman Catholics.

"We practiced rhythm," Tom explained, "but it was very

difficult." Julie had had very irregular cycles all the way from the time when she started having her periods. "It would vary between, say, twenty-eight days up to fifty-five or sixty days," Tom recalled. "Well, we kept track of it. We took her temperature every morning and recorded it versus the day of the cycle. This would give some indication of when ovulation would occur. And, of course, we both looked at this chart. We tried to avoid relations during the period when she would have ovulated and been fertile."

Despite their meticulous record keeping and their careful study of the charts, the result was four more blond, blue-eyed girls in seven years. With such a history, Julie should have acquired the right in her obstetrician's office to be regarded as a human being with a very human problem. Instead, she was just an anonymous white record card. Her doctors were a team of three specialists who shared a suite of offices and a practice. When Julie went to see the doctor, she never knew which one it would be. And when she had a baby, she never knew which one of the three was going to announce, "It's a girl."

Tom described it as "a big assembly line. No one doctor had a real personal relationship with the patient. The patients were kind of rotated among the doctors. It wasn't like going to a family physician. No matter how busy he is, one doctor can look at your record and you can reestablish a relationship and give him a few reminders who you are and what he said the last time."

When Julie made an appointment to see one of the doctors, she pointed out to him that the rhythm method of birth control obviously wasn't working for them because her periods were so extremely irregular. The doctor suggested that she take the Pill. "Julie told him right away that she was a Catholic," Tom said. "And he said, 'Well, I'm giving it to you for medical reasons. I won't prescribe it for you until you go first and tell your priest. Talk to your priest and tell him why I'm giving it.'

"The doctor told her that if she would take the Pill for six months to a year, then after she stopped taking it the cycles would be more regular. He said that the Pill had a tendency to adjust the hormone system of the body in some way so that the cycle became more regular for a goodly period of time after cessation of the Pill."

So Julie "went to Monsignor O'Hara," Tom said, "who was our pastor at the time, and talked with him. He said that it was a strictly medical matter. If [the doctor] was giving it to her for some condition that he felt was necessary from a medical standpoint, why, then she was justified in taking it. Julie called the doctor back after she had seen the priest and the doctor phoned the prescription to the drugstore so we could pick it up."

When we talked to Tom several years after Julie died, he had the baby books for the five children spread out in front of him. "She was an excellent mother," he said. "She thought a tremendous amount about her children and her family life. If you go through these books and see the comments on the pictures and about the children's first prayers and the concern that's reflected anytime there was any sort of illness, you understand that it was more than a bookkeeping job. It really reflects how important the children were to her."

He read some of Julie's comments to us:

"At eighteen months, Anne Marie would fold hands before we said grace at meals.

"At two and a half, she tries to repeat the prayers and make the sign of the cross."

Tom kept leafing through the books. "Here's a picture, for example—'First Birthday Party.' It's a picture I apparently took. She's there holding Kitty in her arms, and underneath it says, 'One candle and look at that yum-yum cake.' And here's another picture showing Kitty being fed the cake."

"Oh, we had plans"

Tom paused and recalled softly, "I remember, I think the most joyful look I ever saw on her face was when our first child, Anne Marie, was born. The nurse brought the baby into the room. It was the first time she saw the baby, you know, and fed it. She had completely recovered from the anesthetic at that time. I never saw such a look of joy on a person's face as I saw that time. It was a reaction she had with each of our little girls. I particularly remember the first time a little bit more because it was the first and it was a tremendous thing for her. I got a little of an understanding of what this means to a woman, that first time, from the expression on her face."

Julie's sister also had vivid memories of the joy Julie found in her children and her husband. "I think her most outstanding characteristic was the love she showed at home; she was a born mother," Peggy said. "Her babies always smelled so sweet. They were healthy and the house was immaculate. She would bring the babies over to our house and I'd pick them up and cuddle them. I would always say, 'Oh, do they smell sweet!' They just did. She kept them so clean."

Tom recalled, "Julie was always happiest when we were working together or doing something as a family.

"One particular incident I remember. We went out and bought one of those outdoor swing sets that were so popular for the backyard. All the kids had to stand around, of course, and watch Daddy put the swing set together. And after it was put together, there was a big rush about who was going to get on first. Lots of giggles and laughs. Of course Mommy and Daddy had to do a little clowning around. I think kids get the greatest kick out of their parents' clowning around.

"I remember I got the camera out and took a few pictures. All sorts of things. And Julie took one of me sliding down the sliding board. I was obviously too big for the sliding board. It's things like this that I remember as our happiest moments, that I keep remembering.

"She was always busy. She liked to knit. Once she was working on a quilt or something. I don't know what you'd call it. It was one of those blankets. It was made up of a large number of individual squares. Each square is knitted with a different pattern. And she did all the mending. We were thinking about buying a sewing machine and had started looking at the different models. . . ."

He paused and shook his head.

"In 1963 we moved into this house. It was September that we moved in and she died just two years later.

"We had so many plans. Naturally, when you're raising five children and you move from a smaller house to a larger house, there's a furniture problem. We used to sit back and plan and say, 'Well, someday we'll have a couch here, and a new rug. We'll get a new dining-room set.' Oh, we had plans. We worked together on putting in a rec room downstairs. We were both very proud of that and were looking forward to furnishing it."

Peggy knew the pride her sister took in the new house and spent many hours talking with her about how it should be furnished as soon as there was enough money. "The sad part of it," Peggy said, "she was just beginning to reap the benefits of all their struggles and sacrifices so that Tom could get his degree. Life was just beginning to be a little more easy. They had a nice home now, but she never lived to see it the way she wanted it."

Julie's life was not an easy one, but it was more than easy. It was satisfying. She knew she was beloved. She knew she was useful. She loved being a mother and a wife and she was a good one. Although their interests were centered in their family, she and Tom also managed to go out and have fun together.

"We live in a neighborhood where people are very close," Tom explained. "We both liked to play bridge. And we'd like to have a night out on the town occasionally to get away from the children. But the family was always Julie's primary interest. All her activities revolved around it. She was active in the Parent-Teacher Association of the parochial school that the older girls attend. And she was very active in church work."

For a time it seemed that Julie and Tom were indeed destined to live happily ever after, but when Julie started taking the Pill to control her menstrual irregularities their life began to change. At first the changes were practically imperceptible. Then they accelerated.

Tom tried to recall exactly what had happened. "Julie would

become very upset and cry. It seemed like it didn't take anything at all to set her off. She would kind of go into a mood and it would last for a day or two.

"And then her attitude toward things changed. She became pessimistic. For example, she would feel that we were in real bad financial shape and that things were not going to improve. They were going to get worse. She used to talk about our financial condition before, but she wouldn't get depressed and pessimistic. Our finances were typical for someone in our position. Naturally we weren't putting a lot of money in the bank or anything like that. But we were paying our bills. There were a lot of time payments, but I think any young married couple with five children has a lot of time payments.

"*All of a sudden* . . ."

"One time during this period, my parents came to visit. I thought Julie would be enthusiastic because she usually was enthused about having them. But she was very depressed. Sometimes, at night particularly, she would just break down and cry. And I'd try to find out why. And there would be no real specific reason for her crying."

Julie was depressed, on and off, for several months. But neither of them connected this change in her normally cheerful disposition with the Pill. Tom was accustomed to doing a fair amount of traveling in connection with his job. Sometimes he would be away just overnight; other times it would be for as long as a week. On the Tuesday before Julie died, he had to go on a trip.

"I returned Friday afternoon and found my wife sick," he told us. "She had been trying to get hold of the doctor. She had called the three rotating physicians, but they couldn't come out to see her.

"She told me she had had several incidents where she would be going about her business and all of a sudden she would get very dizzy and break out in this cold sweat, become pale, and feel very sick. This occurred once when she went shopping, and

I think it happened another time when she went to get her hair fixed. When she went shopping, she had a whole cart full of groceries and she felt so bad, she couldn't even bother with the groceries. She just told the girl to put them back and she got in the car and came home.

"She had been taking bed rest and trying to get hold of a doctor all day. I finally succeeded in getting one to come out Friday night." The doctor checked her over and recommended that she go down to the hospital in the morning so that he could run some tests. He mentioned a chest X ray, blood tests, and a urinalysis.

"The next morning," Tom recalled, "Julie wasn't feeling real well. There were no episodes of this dizziness, though, during the night. When we got ready to go down to the hospital, she wanted me to help her walk. She felt a little unsteady. I was surprised at how weak she was. We got to the hospital about eight-thirty."

The doctor came out to talk to Tom after the tests on Julie had been completed. He seemed cheerful and unconcerned. "He said that he didn't see any reason to admit her to the hospital," Tom said. "The X ray didn't show anything particular. He said something about a broken blood vessel showing up on the X ray, but later on he said, 'I was mistaken about that.'

"He told me there was some pus in the urine and there was some indication of infection. But it wasn't anything that couldn't be cured with bed rest and a little bit of medication."

Julie and Tom could hardly believe their ears—much as they wanted to. Tom had been seriously alarmed at her sudden weakness and Julie couldn't believe she would be feeling so miserable from a little infection. "I thought there was something more serious," Tom said. "And so did my wife. The doctor saw that we were uneasy about it. I said something to the effect that I thought she ought to be admitted to the hospital anyway, or something like that. He came back and said there is nothing in these tests that indicates any reason for having your wife admitted. And I felt a little bit relieved when he said, 'Just bed rest and take this medication. It's just a mild infection.'"

So Tom and Julie went home. He fixed up the sofa in the living room for her with pillows and a blanket and they watched a football game on television together.

"I fixed her a steak, a broiled steak," Tom said. "She ate well."

But she stayed close to the sofa all afternoon. They started watching Jackie Gleason and Julie suddenly became very sick. Tom remembered every moment of it. "She became pale and she broke out in a sweat. She started to breathe real hard. She told me, 'Quick! Call an ambulance!' They arrived fifteen minutes later.

"She asked me to fan her," Tom went on. "She was having trouble getting her breath. And she was white as a sheet, kind of a bluish white, I guess you'd say. And then all of a sudden her chest heaved up and her eyes rolled back in her head and she passed out."

Julie's mother had come over that day to care for the children, and she pitched in, trying to help. For a while she was out on the sidewalk to direct the ambulance to the right house when it came along. Then she joined Tom at the sofa, fanning Julie. Her daughter looked up at her, just before she passed out, and said, "Oh, Mommy, I don't think I'm going to make it."

"The ambulance came," Tom said, "and the driver brought an oxygen bottle in and put her on the stretcher. I held the oxygen on her mouth and we got her to the hospital.

"She was put in the Emergency Room. I was in the waiting room. The doctor came out later. I don't know exactly how much later it was, about forty-five minutes or so. And he said it didn't look too good. And then the nurse came up to him and I could see from the look on her face that she was dead. . . .

"The doctor said, 'I don't understand it. I don't understand it.'"

Tom was not the sort of man who was ready to leave without understanding. He signed the release for an autopsy. And then he made an appointment with a well-recommended internist.

Had Julie died in vain?

The first thing this doctor asked was, "Was she taking birth control pills?"

Tom was surprised. "Yes, does that have anything to do with it?"

"I'll bet," said the doctor, "that the autopsy will show a pulmonary embolism, a thrombus in the ovarian vein."

And he was right. The attending doctor told Tom later that Julie had died from "a thrombus in the right ovarian vein, which caused an embolus which eventually caused the pulmonary embolism."

Tom was not only stunned by the suddenness of Julie's death; he was determined to find out what had really happened. He made a point of researching the effects of the Pill. He read everything relevant that he could get his hands on. He pored over the medical journals and talked to whatever experts were available. He became increasingly convinced that his wife's death had been unnecessary, that just a little time and a little interest would have made the crucial difference as to whether or not the doctor would have prescribed the Pill for medical reasons.

He particularly resented that his wife had not been warned of the dangerous side effects. Slowly, quietly, he became angry. And the more he learned, the angrier he became. "The kind of anger I have," he told us, "I'm not going to run down and throw fire bombs at the office and that kind of thing, but I am angry at what was done, and I think it was wrong."

Tom sued the drug company that had manufactured the particular pill. He lost the case.

The jury of four women and eight men sat for two weeks while pathologists, blood coagulation specialists, gynecologists, and other authorities testified whether or not, in their opinion, the blood clot that killed Julie was unquestionably caused by the Pill. Some of the experts maintained that the clot was indeed Pill-induced; others, testifying for the drug company, dismissed the idea and voiced their opinion that an upper respiratory infection was more likely to have caused Julie's death.

After due deliberation, the jury decided in May 1969 that the manufacturer was not guilty. But this group of responsible men and women had obviously been moved to worry deeply about the medical testimony they had been hearing. Indeed, they had become so concerned that they accompanied their verdict with an unusual and urgent comment. They said that they felt that the manfacturers of this oral contraceptive should make it a regular practice to warn doctors and patients that these pills may be dangerous.

And so, four years after Julie's death, the case was over. Tom had sought $750,000 in damages from the drug company, but to him the money was not principally at stake (although it can be very expensive to bring up five children without a mother). Tom's crusade had been a valiant attempt to ensure that Julie had not died in vain, that her death would become widely known and turn into a warning to other women.

And perhaps it will. The trial was covered by the major news services, and many newspapers sent their own reporters. Reports of the testimony and proceedings appeared in newspapers from coast to coast. (We have changed the names of all the people involved, not because they requested it, but to spare them and particularly the children the emotional upset that might result if friends and neighbors should comment on the very personal details they shared with us.)

Today Tom tries not to look back. His life and that of his daughters is in the future. But it is hard. A family is made of memories and love. He keeps remembering: how they all ate together at the big dining table, the baby in the high chair beside Julie, how they all piled in the car for a week's visit to his folks to show the girls off to the relatives.

He keeps telling people, "She was a real person, the mother of five, not a statistic. And she was an important part—she and a thousand other mothers—of what we call the human race."

Her sister's thoughts deserve to be recorded, too. "What got me the most," Peggy says, "was when I stood at the casket at the funeral. With our faith, I have to think she would go to heaven, but instead I kept thinking to myself—I know she wanted to raise those girls. I can't think that she's really happy being where she is rather than being here."

Peggy stopped for a moment.

"But the saddest thing of all is that, except for the two older girls, I don't think the little girls will remember their mother."

CHAPTER 3

Blood-clotting: Number One Danger

Mrs. Iris J., thirty-nine and married for eighteen years, was posing in front of what was probably the most elaborate and expensive camera in town, the pride of Dr. Elias Rand of Brooklyn. She looked trim in black pants topped with a sunshine-yellow shirt. Her hairdo was fresh and flawless. Rand's assistant, Rose O'Neill, guided Iris into a variety of positions as the giant mobile camera clicked away. It focused on her bosom. She was photographed from the front and from both sides. Then Iris was turned around. Rose guided her into more intricate positions on instructions from the doctor. At one point Iris sat with her left arm twisted around her neck while she seemed to hug the huge camera with her right.

"I'd hate to have to hold this pose for an hour," Iris exclaimed. She didn't have to. Two minutes were enough. Dr. Rand was not interested in her face, her figure, or her clothes. He was doing a lung scan, and it may have saved her life.

Iris had been on the Pill for two months when she developed almost unbearable headaches. Later, there were times when she wheezed. At other occasions she had pains in her chest. Iris had never had headaches before, so she asked her doctor if they might be caused by the Pill.

He said, "No."

Finally the combination of headaches, chest pains, wheezing,

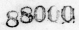

and a general feeling of ill-being pushed her to take further action. She called the county medical society, described her symptoms, and asked for the name of a doctor who could find out what was causing them. They suggested Dr. Rand, who has a radioisotope scanner in his private office, before which Iris was asked to pose. When she called him and described her symptoms, he immediately set up an appointment for her. In cases of such intense headaches, there is always the suspicion that a stroke or other cerebrovascular crisis may be impending. Delay may mean death.

Dr. Rand was able to study Iris's lung scan within a quarter of an hour from the time he had given Iris an injection of radioactive isotopes that raced through her blood so that blood concentrations would show up in the scan. It showed abnormalities in one section of the lung that seemed to indicate that she might have suffered a blood clot there. It did not, however, seem life-threatening at the moment. Dr. Rand felt it was severe enough for him to order her to stop the Pill immediately, to get a lot of rest, and to come in for checkups every week until the diagnosis could be firmly clarified.

The most dramatic part of the checkup was yet to come. Because of the severity and duration of Iris's headaches, Dr. Rand wanted to make certain that there were no areas of major blockage in the brain. He was now going to do a brain scan. Should any abnormalities appear, as in the lung scan, Iris would have to be hospitalized immediately.

We waited tensely while Rose O'Neill posed Iris in front of the giant camera for a second round of scans, this time of her brain. Iris had to wear special glasses so that the eye area would not show up on the picture in a confusing way.

The first shot was ready before she had finished posing for her second set of pictures.

It was normal. This was encouraging but not conclusive. The second and third series of pictures were also normal. We all breathed a sigh of relief. Iris could go home.

Iris is likely to get better with no more trouble. Her symptoms were relieved when she went off the Pill. A highly qualified specialist is supervising her case. With luck, the only long-term effect she will suffer from her three years on the Pill will be her medical bills.

Clots: seeds of death

Every blood clot carries the seeds of death or lifelong illness —and women who take the Pill develop clotting diseases four to eleven times as often as women who do not.

Blood clots were the first side effect of the Pill to be reported, and the first to be accepted by the medical profession.* But today, almost twenty years later, we have no widely accepted test to identify women who are at high risk of developing clots. We know that women with high blood pressure and women over thirty-five run considerably higher risks than others. Some researchers also believe that clotting disorders are related to smoking. Others disagree, however, and the relationship of smoking to clotting and stroke is not as clear-cut as it is to heart disease. Studies published in the *British Medical Journal* in 1977 and the *Annals of Internal Medicine* in 1978 found only weak links between clotting disorders and smoking.

We do not yet have a way to prevent the tragedy of healthy young women dying from Pill-related blood illnesses. One of the most common of these is thrombophlebitis, which means clot formation and inflammation in a vein. Doctors usually cannot tell whether the clot resulted from the vein inflammation or whether the vein inflammation resulted from the clot. That is only the beginning of what doctors don't know about thrombophlebitis. The author of a standard medical textbook on the subject, Dr. J. Edwin Wood, acknowledges that thrombophlebitis is "poorly understood. Two factors are known to be of major importance," Dr. Wood says. They are

* The Pill affects the blood in a number of ways, increasing the risk of clots, heart attacks, and stroke. This chapter deals only with clots of the limbs and lungs; heart attack and stroke are covered in the following two chapters.

"reduced velocity of the flow of the blood . . . and an increase in blood coagulability (thickening)."

The Pill affects both factors. It causes veins to dilate (widen) abnormally, which causes blood to flow more slowly, which in turn may encourage the formation of blood clots. Pill users form blood clots faster than nonusers, and the clots they form are firmer. The Pill also increases the odds that the veins may become varicose in time.

How clots kill

Some women who develop blood clots are lucky. The clot disappears, leaving little or no aftermath. In other cases the clot may permanently impair circulation, usually in the leg but sometimes elsewhere. Surgery may be required. Sometimes the limb itself—or part of it—must be amputated.

What doctors fear most, however, is that a clot may break loose from the vein where it developed and travel. When this happens, the clot becomes an embolus and can be fatal. The most common clotting deaths among Pill users are from clots that originated in the feet, legs, or pelvic region and traveled to the lung.

The Food and Drug Administration now admits that several hundred otherwise healthy young women die each year from Pill-caused clots that travel to the lung. The federal agency also advises women to stop taking the Pill for at least a full cycle before surgery. Because the Pill increases the risk of postoperative clotting complications, patients should also stay off the Pill for at least two weeks after any operation.

New mothers who choose not to nurse their babies should avoid the Pill and similar synthetic hormones, including DES, that are widely used to dry up their milk. These, too, can cause blood clots. Women who take milk-suppressing drugs are three to eight times more likely to develop clots than those who do not.

The drug companies make a great deal of a research study that indicates that the low-dose Pill causes fewer clots than the higher-dose one. This "research," however, is inconclusive. Two other studies, in Manchester, England, and in Walnut Creek, California, show the opposite may be true: changes in the blood that could lead to clots are not related to the amount of the hormone the Pill contains. While it is always advisable to take the lowest effective dose of any medication, the low-dose Pill should not be considered "safe."

There are no valid figures available to tell us either how many women have been treated for blood clots by doctors at home or how many have been hospitalized for clotting disorders. No one knows how many Pill users may be walking around this minute with undetected or unnoticed clots, although the experts guess that the figure may be high.

Clotting disorders can sometimes be detected before there is pain, swelling, or any other symptom. These "silent" thrombi (or clots) can be found in laboratory analysis of blood samples. Researchers in the United States found these silent clots among a group of 154 women who were tested before they started the Pill and again three months later. Clots were four to five times as common after the Pill had been taken. A team of British researchers came to the same conclusion while testing for thrombosis in surgical patients. Six out of 31 Pill users had silent clots, but none of 19 women who did not use the Pill had this problem.

Responsible doctors are concerned about the Pill not only because it may trigger disabling or deadly traveling blood clots, but also because once a woman has developed even a relatively minor clot of this type, the chances are 50 percent or higher that she will develop other clots. And each one carries the seed of death.

Alice B. was hospitalized in 1973 with a clot in her leg; her doctor recognized the clot as a side effect of the Pill. In 1977, after Alice had been off the Pill for four years, her leg became swollen and painful again, the result of another bout of thrombophlebitis. Alice spent several weeks at home with her feet up and seems to have recovered. She has regular checkups, including tests for the clotting factors in her blood. Alice takes care of herself and hopes for the best, but she will live with the fear of another, potentially deadly, clot for the rest of her life.

Alice, however, was lucky as clot victims define the word *lucky*. For once the clotting process starts, it can be difficult to control, as the following two cases illustrate.

Betty H. and Anita A. headed straight for New York City when they graduated from college. Bright and attractive, they became the center of one of the many sets of singles in the city. Anita started graduate school at New York University and, much to her delight, almost immediately embarked on a love affair with one of her professors, a married man. Betty got a job as a caseworker with the Welfare Department and fell in love with Leon, a fellow caseworker.

The two young women went to a family planning clinic for contraceptive advice. Each girl saw a different doctor. Both doctors recommended the Pill. They did not even discuss alternative methods of contraception, a fact that did not bother Betty or Anita. Women who were "with it" were also "with" the Pill.

Three months after Betty started the Pill, she developed painful clots in both legs and in her left arm. She was taken off the Pill, hospitalized, and treated with heparin, a powerful anticoagulant that can be administered only in a hospital. Upon her release from the hospital, the doctor placed her on Coumadin, a milder anticoagulant, and instructed her to wear a waist-high elastic stocking that has the approximate "give" of a firm girdle and helps maintain normal blood flow.

"It's a terrible nuisance," Betty said. "Sometimes it takes me almost an hour to ease on in the morning and almost as long to get off at night. You always feel terribly hot and sweaty. And it looks terrible."

Leon visited Betty every evening in the hospital, brought her flowers, and thought up little surprises to amuse her. But once she got home, the love affair ground to a halt. Betty was weak. It was all she could do to get through her work. And Leon, as Betty said, was "just not a Robert Browning. He didn't want to sit around and read me poetry all night while I kept my legs elevated. He wanted to go out and have fun or stay in and have sex. And I wasn't up to doing either one."

Despite the drug therapy and the elastic stocking, the clots in her legs became worse again and Betty had to go back to the hospital for intensive treatment with heparin. Shortly after she was dismissed, at least one clot (and perhaps several) moved to her lung. She had to go back to the hospital for a third time. More clots traveled to the lung. Now the doctors decided that surgery was necessary.

Betty recovered from this major surgery and has been back at work for almost two years. She is still under close medical supervision, still wears the detestable elastic stocking, still is on and off anticoagulants. Her doctors describe her as "chronically incapacitated." There have been no men in her life since Leon walked out of it. Her job, her trips to the doctor, and her daily struggle with the elastic stocking shape her life and she sees no hope for change.

Anita's first clot did not develop until she had been on the Pill for twenty-eight months. Conforming to a pattern that has become all too familiar since the advent of the Pill, she developed other clots, all in the right leg, and has had to be hospitalized four times. Like Betty, she is on and off blood-thinning drugs as well as in and out of Ace bandages. When Anita's clots flare up, her leg becomes hot, sore, and swollen.

"I take much more Darvon [a pain-killing drug] than I should," Anita says, "but I just can't stand it. It's not only the pain," she continued, "it's that once you know you have it you're always frightened. There's a cloud hanging over you.

"I was in the hospital," she said, "when I saw the newspaper reports about the English doctors who established a definite relationship between blood clots and the Pill. I've never had the urge to kill before, but if that damn doctor who first gave me the Pill had been standing in the room, I think I would have leaped out of bed and strangled him.

"Even when I feel okay, I never know when I'll have a flare-up. I have to think about it all the time. I can't sit in one position too long. I can't exercise or risk getting too tired. When the clots are bad, I'm not allowed to drive. Even when they don't bother me, I can't drive for more than an hour.

"I don't think my life has ever really been in danger," Anita told us, "but it's been one big mess. I'm twenty-eight years old and I want to start enjoying my youth before it's all over. I've finally decided to go ahead with surgery. It's an elective procedure called vein stripping." (This involves removal of the vein or veins with the clots and it is not always effective.)

While Betty is sadly resigned to her condition and Anita is angry, Mrs. Rose L., who lives in a small town in South Dakota, is philosophical. She was in her early thirties when she developed her incapacitating leg clot. With the encouragement of one of her doctors, she brought suit against the company that manufactured the birth control pill she had taken and received a substantial out-of-court settlement.

"What is to be is to be," Mrs. L. believes. "What happened to me is God's will. Maybe God did this to me so I could help other women and warn them about the terrible things this pill can do to a person's body. If my story makes one person stop taking the Pill," Mrs. L. wrote us, "I'll be happy."

Here is an account of Mrs. L.'s experience in her own words:

"Now all I had heard about the Pill was that it made you as sick as when you are pregnant. And I was very sick with all three children so I sure didn't want that. So I asked my doctor, 'Can it hurt me in any way?'

"He said, 'No. Not in any way.' So I started taking it. It did make me a little nauseated for the first few days, but that was okay."

"The pain was awful"

"On the nineteenth day, I had been sitting and talking on the phone when I got up and took about ten steps. This awful cramp, like sharp pain, hit my upper leg in the back and I couldn't move. I wanted to call for help, but my husband was outside in the car waiting for me. The cramp sort of let up and I could move. I had to limp a little. It hurt!

"I went on the rest of the day and kept off of it some. When I lay down and put it up, it wouldn't hurt so bad. By the second day lying down didn't help. I figured I had arthritis. I took aspirin and I carried on.

"In the meanwhile I took the rest of the pills. On the third day, we took our boy to his doctor because he had a sore throat. That doctor noticed that I was limping when I came in and asked to look at me.

"I told him about the leg and he just felt it and then asked, 'Have you been taking the Pill?' I told him, 'Yes.' He was sort of angry and said something about 'some doctors.' He told me, 'You have a very large blood clot. You must get it cut out right away or you will die.'

"I phoned the clinic and told the receptionist, 'I just came from a doctor and he told me I had a blood clot.'

"Her first words were, 'Are you taking the Pill? Don't take any more of them.' Then I talked to the nurse and she used the very same words. I was told to get to the clinic quickly.

"In the hospital, the first day I started on some drugs and X rays, I couldn't even let one foot out of bed. I was taking lots of medication every day and had my blood checked every day. I was there for twenty-eight days. I was so worried about my three kids. My poor husband had to cook for the kids, keep the washing done, and come see me. The kids hung up the wash and did the dishes and swept the floors.

"After I got home from the hospital, I had to have my blood checked every day, then every two days, then once a week. I was on so many pills! The pain was awful.

"I can't tell you what my husband went through or what he felt. I would scream at him for no reason. I moaned in my sleep and was terrified that he would bump my leg in the night. Our sex life was the same way. My leg was so sore that it would hurt for five full minutes from just a touch.

"For four months I went to the clinic every week. A blood test, then up to see Dr. T. and he would tell me how great I was. Then to Dr. M. and get my medicine.

"The doctor lets me wear an elastic hip stocking with a long-legged girdle. I still have to take nerve pills and sometimes pain pills. I can't run, jump, or go on long walks or swim. My clothes fit one day, and maybe the next day if I am swelled up I can't even get in them. My shoe is the same way.

"I can dance a little and do a fair day's work if I rest a lot.

"I hate to see the wrinkles on my face like an old lady, but pain puts them there and it keeps them there. My face looks like my mother's and she is fifty-nine."

Rose L. came perilously close to losing her leg. Susan T. did lose her leg. She had been on the Pill for thirty-one days when she developed severe pain and swelling in her left leg. It happened very quickly. The leg had been swollen for a few days, but she had hardly taken notice of it because her mother had been extremely ill. She was in the hospital visiting her mother when the pain suddenly became so intense that she called a nurse.

Susan was admitted to the hospital on the spot as an emergency patient. The following day, surgery was performed and a large number of blood clots were discovered. Efforts to remove or reduce them proved futile. The circulation in the leg came to a halt. A few days later, gangrene developed and the leg was removed below the knee. It turned out that even this surgery was not enough. Moist gangrene developed in the upper portion of the leg, and it had to be removed also. Two years have passed, and Susan T., a housewife with one young child, is struggling to get accustomed to her artificial leg. She can't stoop down to scrub a bathtub or clean the oven. She can't handle a broom and dustpan. She can't turn a mattress. Susan T. is just now learning how to make a bed again.

A neat, attractive brunette, who used to be a bookkeeper before her marriage, Susan rarely goes out socially now. She and her husband live in a small town. There isn't anyplace much to go except for the movies, but she still finds it too difficult to get in and out of the closely ranged seats in the local theater.

Since Susan's trouble, the general practitioner in her town has taken considerable pains to translate the technical product information that comes with each of the various birth control pills into simple English for laypersons. Now when a woman asks him for the Pill, he hands her his "translation" and tells her, "If you want to take it, this is what can happen." If a woman persists in wanting the Pill, he tells her the story of Susan.

Women came to suspect the Pill by watching, and hearing about, other women who suffered from its "rare" side effects. In many cases they were far ahead of their doctors in recognizing how dangerous this drug is.

Mrs. Alma J. is a secretary with three grown children who lives in a suburb of Stockholm, Sweden. When she was forty-three, she began to be troubled by irregular and painful menstruation. She visited her private doctor and was given a prescription for the Pill.

She began to take it two weeks before her daughter was to be married. On the fourteenth day, the day before the wedding, she got a blood clot in her left foot and another in her right hand. Neither she, nor her doctor, who treated her, were convinced there could be any connection between the Pill and the clots, but she was taken off oral contraceptives.

A year later she had the same painful menstrual trouble. This time she went to the Women's Clinic at the famous Karolinska Hospital in Stockholm. The doctor there said she should take the Pill. Alma told him she would prefer to have some other type of medication and related what had happened the previous time. The doctor and nurses laughed at her and said there could be no connection between the blood clots and the Pill.

She reluctantly accepted the prescription, got the pills, and began to take them. Fourteen days later she got another thrombosis in the leg.

Later, when she angrily told the doctor at Karolinska what the Pill had done, he laughed once again and said there could be no connection. Alma then wrote about her "case" in a letter to Professor Erik Ask-Upmark, about whose studies she had read. He replied gratefully that she was undoubtedly right about the cause of her blood clots, and sent her a bunch of flowers.

When we related this case to Dr. Barbro Westerholm of the Swedish Committee on Adverse Reactions she told us: "This is the classic way of confirming a relationship. Of course we can't deliberately try to provoke a thrombosis in a woman a second time. But when you want evidence of a causative agent, this is how you get it."

Thirty-one Christmases

Gillian N., who had a pulmonary embolism, was admitted to a large midwestern hospital on December 18. On the night of December 22, her husband, Michael, brought the two children to visit her, Kevin, five, and Sandra, who was almost eight. Kevin gave her a big hug and asked her if she would be home for Christmas. Gillian told her son that she wasn't sure, but she'd try. Gillian was not able to get home for Christmas. She died on Christmas Eve.

Shortly before Thanksgiving, Gillian, who was thirty-one, had had a pain in her left calf. She went to her doctor, who told her that she might have pulled a ligament and that she should take it easy for a few days. The pain got worse, however, and she went back. "You might have a superficial blood clot," he told her, "but it's nothing to get alarmed about. Keep your leg elevated and keep hot towels on it. Incidentally, I see that I gave you a prescription for birth control pills last August. You'd better stop taking them, at least until this clears up."

Gillian followed the doctor's instructions, but the pain continued and spread to her left thigh and then the left side of her abdomen. Her leg grew increasingly swollen and discolored. "It was purplish when she came in," says Helen, who was Gillian's hospital roommate.

Gillian's husband was a policeman. She worked part-time as a bookkeeper to supplement the family income. They needed the money badly, and for the first week of her illness Gillian tried to work at home. After that she was too weak and miserable to do anything.

When she began to complain of strong pains in what she described as the area of her heart, the doctor hurried her into the hospital.

Helen, who was recovering from gallbladder surgery—and who did get home for Christmas—liked Gillian right off. "She set her hair every night," Helen said, "so she would look nice for her husband. She tried to cooperate with the nurses. I could tell that she wasn't getting better, though. She would roll over sometimes and you could hear her quietly moaning and kind of curling up and holding her stomach, but she never complained. You could tell that she was worried.

"The first time she passed out was about three days before she died. She had tests and things almost every day and she was on this very strict diet. They stopped giving her pills for pain and gave her shots instead.

"Toward the end, even I could tell she was in extremely serious condition. She was having trouble breathing and was screaming, out of her mind with pain. It was the worst thing I have ever seen. Once, just before she passed out, she was lying back, and her eyes were closed, and she said, 'Helen, call the nurse.' And she opened her eyes and her eyes were rolling back in her head.

"It was evident that she was getting worse. She winced a lot and lay there and closed her eyes like she was trying to bear it without hollering. I don't know if you would call it white or gray, but she would turn color and take terrible deep breaths. She didn't want the covers on and they kept putting them back on. You could hear her trying to gulp air and she couldn't. She would try it and then kind of fall back again like she couldn't make it.

"When she lay dying the doctor came in and I heard him say, 'Oxygen. And quick.' It took quite a while, but she did begin to breathe. They were great, big, horrible, shuddering breaths like she was trying to get in all the air she could possibly get hold of. I've never been able to forget it."

"The morning of Christmas Eve, she started to scream. Practically every five minutes. Then it was just one continuous horrible scream after another. She kept asking for her husband and her mother and then later on there was nothing. She didn't say anything more. She was dying in all this agony and pain. Why couldn't they do something for her in this modern hospital?"

Gillian, the wife and mother who saw only thirty-one Christmases. And why? Because the Pill that is supposed to be such a boon to women, to help them escape the trap of their own fertility, betrayed its promise. Gillian escaped the fertility trap, but not the death trap. Did the doctors, residents, and interns who followed Gillian's case and heard her screams change their minds about the Pill? We don't know.

We do know of one doctor in Danbury, Connecticut, who became extremely cautious about prescribing the Pill after treating Mrs. Dawn McK. He referred Mrs. McK. to us because he thought her story might make other women—and physicians—change their minds about the desirability of oral contraceptives. Mrs. McK. suffered from the beginning with coughing, tiredness, chest pains, and headaches.

"The headaches happened with each period, the first two days. They were fierce. Aspirin didn't help, or Bufferin or Darvon. My husband wanted me to stop the Pill, but the doctor said, 'Well, go along with it for a while.'

"In March I started getting a pain in the back of my chest. Also a slight cough if I was overtired. I called the doctor and he did a chest X ray. It showed nothing. We went along like this until August 12, the day I went into the hospital.

"That morning I gave the house a good cleaning. At eight-forty, I went into a restaurant next to the store where I work and had some coffee. When I tried to get off the stool at the restaurant I couldn't feel the floor. I barely made it next door. I said to my boss, 'Catch me. I'm passing out.'"

A traveling clot had blocked a large blood vessel in her lung.

"I lay perfectly still in the hospital for the next two months. When I left, I kept on taking blood-thinning pills until April 20 and I went to the hospital once a week for a blood test.

"I'll never forget the day the doctor came to my room. His face was white. 'I have another case almost exactly like yours,' he told me, 'but she's not taking it as well.'

"The week I got out of the hospital I read about a girl in Bridgeport, twenty-three years old, who died from a pulmonary embolism like I had. Then I realized why the doctor kept telling me, 'You're a very lucky girl.'

"One of my neighbors, she has, I mean she had, a girl my daughter's age—she was twenty-nine. She died from the Pill a few months ago. They said it was a clot in the brain. She was having bad headaches, but she didn't know about the danger of headaches. Now I always tell my experience to anyone who's having headaches, even though I'm so ashamed of having taken the Pill. I can never go to confession with a clear mind. My priest doesn't know. One of these days I'll get up the courage to tell him. And soon I'll have to tell my daughters. I *must* tell my daughters," Dawn said with great distress. "My daughter-in-law, too. I must protect them from harm. But I'm so afraid they will say, 'Wasn't she terrible to take the Pill?'"

We hope they won't. We don't think Dawn did a terrible thing in taking the Pill. The Pill did a terrible thing to her.

CHAPTER 4

Heart Disease and the Pill

The Pill alters so many basic bodily functions that researchers had long suspected that it could cause heart attacks and cardiovascular illness. But it took almost fifteen years for the first definitive research to prove the association between heart attacks and the Pill. In 1975 and 1976 two British researchers, J. I. Mann and W. H. W. Inman, published a series of papers showing that Pill users had three to five times more risk of heart attack than other women.

The finding came as no surprise to specialists in the Pill's effects on metabolism. They had long known that the Pill tended to shift a woman's tolerance of sugar (toward diabetes), raise her blood pressure, and build up the fat deposits in her blood. Each of these changes, by itself, would raise her risk of a heart attack; but each change is subtle, and each may be just the start of what can be a long period before actual disease develops.

Dr. William N. Spellacy is one of the world's leading authorities on how the Pill affects metabolism. His research, which was supported by the Food and Drug Administration, began in 1962 but is now severely curtailed because of an unexplained cut in that funding. He told us that "the Pill produces changes in growth hormone, carbohydrate [sugar] metabolism, and lipid [fat] metabolism, which are tied together." When a woman is on the Pill, "even the amino acids in meat are metabolized differently. It appears that the incidence of abnormalities in the blood is related to the length of time a woman has been on the Pill. At five years you get fewer abnormal tests than at ten years. In most people there isn't much real abnormality before two years. You get chemical changes, but you don't get real abnormal values."

One of the consequences of the Pill that Dr. Spellacy considers a "major change" is a rise in triglyceride levels in the blood. Triglycerides are associated with hardening of the arteries and with heart disease.

The entire picture of the blood in women who have been on the Pill for several years is such that even in the 1960s some investigators, such as Dr. William R. Hazzard of the Veterans Administration Hospital in Seattle, asked whether the Pill may deprive women of one advantage that they have over men: their ability to resist coronary disease (heart attacks), especially in middle age.

At a symposium on drugs affecting lipid metabolism held in Milan, Italy, Dr. Colin H. Bolton, a biochemist at Radcliffe Infirmary in Oxford, England, declared, "When women take oral contraceptives, the behavior of their platelets [disks in the blood that are concerned with clotting] resembles that of patients with arterial disease." Dr. Bolton said this was "apparently due to the estrogen component of the oral contraceptives."

Changes in blood fats

Dr. Russell R. de Alvarez of Temple University in Philadelphia, also investigated the Pill's impact upon fat metabolism. In evaluating various brands of the Pill and the changes in fat metabolism produced by each, Dr. de Alvarez found that those containing the greatest amount of estrogen in proportion to progestin caused the most pronounced changes in fat metabolism.

Later research both confirms and confuses his findings. The

level of estrogen in each brand of the Pill seems to have an effect on the blood fats, but so does the level of the progestin component. As of late 1979, the most anyone could say was that each brand had a unique effect, depending upon the balance of its hormones. But there is no pill available that will not increase fat levels in the blood. One pill (Norinyl 1+50) raises blood cholesterol less than the others tested; the researchers concluded that the rise in cholesterol was "insignificant" for this pill, although more important for the others.

Back in 1969 Dr. John J. Schrogie, who was then the principal expert on oral contraceptives for the Food and Drug Administration, summed up the situation as follows: "It's a confluence of factors which seem to be coming together at the same time. We have a situation where the changes in lipid [fat] metabolism are going in the same direction, in essence, as the changes in carbohydrate [sugar] metabolism. If you add changes in coagulation [blood-clotting] activity on top of this, what can be created here is a fairly high risk of premature cardiovascular disease."

In other words, the effect of the Pill on the heart is not a great unknown but a proven risk.

Blood pressure, too

There is another underlying risk factor in heart disease, hypertension, or high blood pressure that is also affected by the Pill. Several studies have now proved that most women who decide to take the Pill will have a small rise in their blood pressure, and a small but significant number of them will develop hypertension. The increased pressure seems to occur in the vast majority of women who take oral contraceptives. Women who have suffered from hypertension during pregnancy do not develop it more often than others when they start on the Pill. The increase in blood pressure continues the longer the Pill is used; a study performed by the Royal College of General Practitioners in England showed that hypertension was two to two and one-half times as common among women who had taken the Pill for five years. Blood pressure usually drops back to normal, or slightly below normal, when the Pill is discontinued, but it remains elevated in a small percentage of women.

Hypertension, by itself, can be a painful and disabling disease and can lead to death. In some cases the pressure on the blood vessels becomes so great that a vein or an artery bursts and the patient may die. High blood pressure often, however, leads to coronary disease, creating such a strain on the heart that it stops functioning.

As long ago as January 23, 1965, an article appeared in the *British Medical Journal* reporting the case of a hitherto healthy thirty-three-year-old woman who, after three years on the Pill, died of a coronary thrombosis. The doctor reporting the incident asked, "Is there an increased risk of coronary thrombosis in taking the Pill? And, if so, are we justified in subjecting our patients to this risk?"

In 1966, the British journal *Lancet* carried reports expressing concern over the effects of the Pill on the heart from as far away as Sweden and Ghana. Swedish researchers reported in February of that year, and again the following December, that "during administration of oral contraceptives" certain fats in the blood of young women change and assume patterns similar to those seen in postmenopausal women and in men, indicating an increased susceptibility to coronary disorders.

A report from Ghana along the same worrying line suggested that "the protective value of the female endocrine system against development of early cardiovascular atherosclerotic disease may be seriously impaired by use of oral contraceptives." The report also expressed concern over changes in Pill users' mineral metabolism,* especially of magnesium, and pointed out that a high magnesium intake helps protect the hearts of rats against the ravages of high-cholesterol diets.

---

* See Chapter 14 for a discussion of these and other nutritional effects.

"She was dead"

These reports did not, however, save Mrs. Joyce C., who lived in a large city of the English Midlands. Joyce, aged thirty-three, had lost one child who was stillborn. At Joyce's inquest, a neighbor testified: "This upset her and she wanted no further pregnancies in case the same thing happened again. She already had one son, aged twelve years. On May 29 she called at my house after coming home from work at dinnertime. She was complaining of a tightness in her chest. I gave her a cup of tea and she then went home. At 3:00 P.M. she came back again and asked for help, as she felt very ill and had bad pains in her chest. I helped her onto my bed and then telephoned for Dr. B."

The doctor, recalling that Joyce "was terrified of any further pregnancies," testified that in January he "prescribed four months' supply of the contraceptive pill. . . . In May I took her off these pills and gave her four months' supply of another type of birth pill, as she was complaining of some discomfort in her breasts and was putting on weight.

"There was no further record of her coming for another supply of pills until two years later, when she came to see me again. She wanted to start taking contraceptive pills again, so I prescribed to her six months' supply of a newer type of pill. She was to take twenty-one per month. Three months later, I was asked to go and see her. I saw her at 3:40 P.M. and she was complaining of chest pains. I realized that she had had a very severe coronary thrombosis and gave her an injection of one-half grain of morphia. I then went to phone for an ambulance. When I returned, she was dead. In my experience, I have never heard of a young woman having a coronary. . . ."

When we called on Joyce's physician, the thin-lipped, candid Dr. B., the following year, he was still shaken.

"Every time I write out a prescription for the Pill," he told us, "I get an emotional shock. Yes, I still write them, but never without thinking of Joyce. I can never forget the words of that pathologist's report.

"After thirty years in the practice of medicine, of course, there are many hard, hurting memories. But I think that day was one of the saddest in my whole professional life. As soon as I got to the house and saw Joyce, I knew I was seeing an acute coronary attack, though it was difficult to believe that it could be happening to a girl just past thirty. I just stood there, helpless. Her twelve-year-old son came home from school. I had to tell him. He couldn't believe it, that his mother was dead. I waited until Joyce's husband could get home from work."

"You actually waited at the house?"

"Of course. It was the least I could do."

What about patients who want contraceptive advice from Dr. B. today? He said that he explained the whole female cycle to them, told them about all methods, and then waited to see what their reactions were.

"Most women are quite aware that there have been deaths attributed to the Pill. They also understand that I cannot tell them whether they—as individuals—are likely to become a sad statistic, excluding, of course, the women for whom there are definite contraindications, such as a previous thromboembolic experience. Those women I can tell quite certainly: 'You shouldn't be on the Pill.' But the rest—well, I have to let them make their own choice."

Like Joyce, Beatrice S., a thirty-seven-year-old housewife in Liverpool, England, who died when a clot that her doctor believed was triggered by the Pill struck the arteries that supply her heart, was also "fortunate" in a way. She died with merciful speed.

Beatrice had been on the Pill for about three months, her husband told the coroner. "She took them every evening after dinner. She complained that they made her tired, but that didn't alarm her since many of her friends had the same experience. The doctor at the family planning clinic told her that it might take several months to adapt to them.

"She was on her way to collect the children from nursery

school," her husband reported, "when she collapsed and was brought home by taxi. Doris, our neighbor, put her to bed. She started to improve. The next day I went to work at eight-fifteen. She was sitting up in bed and seemed better."

Doris dropped in shortly after ten o'clock the next morning to see how Beatrice was doing. "When I got into her bedroom," Doris told the coroner, "she was bent forward in a jack-knife position. I said, 'How are you?' and she looked up and said, 'Fainting.' I went to fetch some water and when I came back she had collapsed backwards. Then she said, 'Can't breathe. Can't breathe.' I raised her up. She fell back and died."

Unpredictable consequences

Swedish researchers were among the first to warn of possible Pill effects among women with a pronounced family history of heart disease. Dr. Kim Cramer of Sahlgrenska Hospital in Göteborg, who has been studying the effect of the Pill on phospholipids, cholesterol, and other factors in the blood, said: "Women who have a hereditary disposition toward heart and artery diseases should not be burdened with a substance that increases the risk. I share the opinion of other Swedish researchers that we are giving hundreds of thousands of women a form of therapy whose consequences we are unable to foresee."

This conservative approach has not yet been adopted here in the United States. Current drug company literature cautions only that any patient with "cardiac dysfunction" must be carefully observed while on the Pill. Her family history is apparently unimportant to the Pill manufacturers, although the Pill is known to increase the risk of heart trouble.

One of the greatest disappointments and ironies of the Pill was brought out at the 134th annual meeting of the Tennessee Medical Association. The head of the department of obstetrics and gynecology at Vanderbilt University explained that the very women who should avoid becoming pregnant for medical reasons—for instance, women with heart trouble—are also women who should never take the Pill. They are most at risk, because the Pill is too likely to "aggravate their condition." Drs. Celia Oakley and Jane Somerville from the Royal Postgraduate Medical School, Hammersmith Hospital, and the London Institute of Cardiology, reported in the *Lancet* on three women with heart conditions who took the Pill. One died, and the other two were never able to resume their normal lives.

The first case was that of an unmarried woman who died at the age of twenty-four. The two women doctors reported: "A heart murmur had been heard at the age of nine months. Occasional dyspnoea [difficulty in breathing] and cyanosis [blueness of the skin] after effort was noted in childhood. She grew up normally and at age fifteen, her physical signs suggested a large . . . defect. . . . The patient remained well, able to walk any distance, dance and do a full-time job." The girl really did not feel incapacitated. In fact, she considered herself so well that she decided against an extensive examination suggested by the doctor. Three years later, she was examined again and found to be unchanged.

"In November," the doctors wrote, "she came asking for help as she had suddenly become more breathless and tired. She was worried because her friends said she was bluer." The doctors checked her over and suggested that she come back for a more intensive examination. "Owing to family problems, she did not come into hospital for reinvestigation until February," fifteen months later, when she was found to be in very poor condition. Approximately five weeks later she died.

The doctors suggested that the birth control Pill might have caused the rapid worsening of this condition. It turned out that an oral contraceptive had been prescribed to control a menstrual irregularity during the summer before her first visit to seek help. It was considered very suggestive that in May the young woman stated that she felt very well and that it was November of that same year when she came in asking for help.

The doctors pointed out: "There was no pregnancy, trauma, or infection, nor had the patient lived at high altitude—which might have accounted for the change in her . . . state."

Another case cited by the two women doctors was of "a married woman, age twenty-one, with a [heart] defect, [who had] been born by forceps delivery. Her birth weight was seven pounds, three ounces. . . . She was difficult to feed and slow to gain weight in her first year. A heart murmur was first noticed at the age of two years.

"Although she remained underweight with a tendency to respiratory infections, she was active and otherwise symptom-free throughout her childhood and adolescence. . . . She was first seen at Hammersmith Hospital at the age of thirteen years. At that time she could play two sets of tennis. . . . She was a small, thin, intelligent girl. . . ."

"She had become blue . . ."

Examination showed signs of "a big ventricular defect" and "enlarged heart." The electrocardiogram was also abnormal. A few years later, the doctors felt that they could perform surgery to correct the girl's "ventricular defect," but the patient "wanted to get married and to defer cardiac surgery until later." Accordingly, in May she was started on an oral contraceptive pill. Shortly afterward she had two transient attacks of diplopia (double vision) and was changed to another brand of pill. In December . . . she and her family noticed that she had become blue and she herself noticed that she felt tired and unwell. "Four months later . . . the change in her appearance was striking. . . . She was seen to become very breathless after mild effort." The doctors concluded: "Oral contraceptives were stopped, but there was no change in her clinical condition. . . . Since that time there has been no change in the patient's cardiac state—neither reversion to the previous situation nor continuation of the progressive deterioration which had taken place after she had started taking the oral contraceptives."

The third case was of a twenty-year-old married woman with a persistent heart condition that had never really bothered her. Sometimes she became short of breath, such as when she played hockey at school at the age of fourteen. "She remained active and well . . . able to manage a full-time job, shopping, dancing and all routine housework. In June . . . she married and started taking [an oral contraceptive]. In August, she noted increasing dyspnoea [difficulty in breathing]—which surprised her as she had lessened her activities after marriage. Slowly the dyspnoea worsened, and by October she could do nothing in the house and was restricted to a completely sedentary life.

"After having been confined to bed by breathlessness for several weeks she was admitted to the hospital with a long list of serious heart symptoms and intensive treatment was begun.

"Some improvement occurred," the doctors reported. "The patient was discharged and advised not to continue with the contraceptive pill. She required therapy to maintain her improvement, but she never returned to the state of well being present in May. . . ." It was in June that this young woman had started taking the Pill.

As of early 1980, researchers are agreed that the Pill increases the risk of heart attack; they do not agree on how great the risk is. Various studies have shown that women who take the Pill are anywhere from two to fourteen times as likely to have coronary attacks. The degree of risk an individual faces depends upon whether any other factors apply that would predispose her to heart problems: smoking, obesity, poor glucose tolerance, high blood pressure, high fat levels in the blood, or a history of other blood diseases. The Pill contributes to each of these risk factors, with the exception of smoking.

A word about cigarettes

Oral contraceptives and cigarettes seem to act synergistically: that is, they multiply each other's risks, posing special hazards of heart attack for those who use both. The synergistic effect is so strong that women over thirty-five or forty who smoke and use the Pill are almost courting heart disease.

Some doctors feel that for nonsmokers the risks of the Pill are insignificant. This is simply not true.

In a study by Oxford University's Dr. Martin Vessey in 1977, involving over 88,000 women-years of observation, nine women died of cardiovascular diseases. Five of them smoked; four did not. The Royal College study in 1977 reported that, even after standardization for smoking habits, age, social class, and number of children, Pill users are twice as likely to die from vascular diseases as nonusers between twenty-five and thirty-four, and four and one-half times as likely to die between thirty-five and forty-four. Similarly, the data from the long-term British studies has been analyzed statistically by Anrudh K. Jain of the Population Council in New York City. He calculates that among nonsmokers the risk of one kind of heart attack (myocardial infarction) is increased by 50 percent in the thirty-to-thirty-nine group and slightly less than 50 percent in older women. Researchers H. Frederikson and R. T. Ravenholt of the Agency for International Development have estimated that for clotting disorders the incidence jumps almost twenty-three times for those who smoke and use the Pill. But for those who take oral contraceptives and do not smoke the risk is still more than seven times greater.

While the statistical evidence of a synergistic effect between smoking and Pill use is very strong, there are no generally accepted medical explanations. One reason may be that smoking and the Pill have certain effects that are similar.

Both the Pill and smoking, for example, raise blood pressure. Cigarettes, like the Pill, may raise the level of fats in the blood. Smoking, in addition, reduces the amount of oxygen available to the heart and other muscles; oxygen becomes tied up in the blood with the carbon monoxide the smoker inhales. At the same time, smoking increases the heart's need for oxygen by increasing its activity. It is easy to see how these factors might combine to put enormous pressure on the heart.

CHAPTER 5

Strokes and the Pill

Doctors group clotting disorders, heart conditions, and strokes together as circulatory or vascular diseases, and a substantial body of research implicates the Pill as a cause of all three.

The Royal College of Physicians in London estimates that women on the Pill die from diseases of the blood vessels almost five times as often as nonusers. They found that those who had given up the Pill carried it with them in terms of their susceptibility to these diseases. Women who took the Pill and then stopped it were still more than four times as likely to die from vascular disease as those who had never used it. Both this and another British study, that of the Oxford Family Planning Association, confirmed that older women and women who smoke run the greatest risks from the use of oral contraceptives.

Stroke is the third-ranking killer in the United States, after heart attack and cancer, and the second greatest crippler. A stroke, or CVA (cerebrovascular accident), as doctors call it, is essentially the death of a part of the brain. The human brain accounts for only 2 percent of the body's total weight, yet so complex are its functions that it uses one quarter of all the oxygen we breathe. If part of the brain is deprived of its normal supply of oxygen-bearing blood for even a few minutes, that part may die forever, with crippling aftereffects. Depending on the area affected, the person may die.

Strokes tend to be closely related to age. The incidence and risk soar after age sixty. When younger women have strokes, they usually have a specific disease—diabetes or high blood pressure, for instance—that helps explain the "accident." In some cases, stroke appears to be "hormone-dependent." It occurs in connection with pregnancy or the postpartum period when the balance of hormones is temporarily shifted.

In a Pill-taker, a stroke may be due to a blood clot that travels to the brain, or it may be caused by one or more of the underlying bodily changes associated with the Pill. (See Chapter 4 on heart disease.)

Neurologists began to report strokes "from no apparent cause" in otherwise healthy young women shortly after the Pill came into use on a large scale. These cases seemed to have one common denominator: the young women were all on the Pill. The first such case to appear in the medical literature was reported in the *British Medical Journal* in 1962. Now stroke is recognized as a side effect of the Pill.

In September 1968, a group of pathologists, Drs. John H. Altshuler, Roy A. McLaughlin, and Karl T. Neuberger of Denver, Colorado, wrote in the *Archives of Neurology*: "The possibility of a relationship between oral contraceptives and neurologic disease has been under discussion since about 1961. Autopsy studies of pertinent neurological cases, however, have been scarce, especially in this country." The pathologists went on to report their autopsy findings in a case that they considered significant: that of a twenty-six-year-old who was in good health except for a history of mild migraine headaches.

The doctors cited much technical detail from their autopsy to support their conclusion that this young woman's "neurological catastrophe," or stroke, was linked to the Pill. Explaining why he is quite certain that the Pill led to her death, one of the pathologists, Dr. Neuberger, said: "It was a very unusual combination of findings. The changes in the blood vessels that you see in older stroke victims or the findings associated with injury or illness were not present in this case. There was no other cause."

Similar deaths have been reported all over the world. In approximately one quarter of the cases there is apparently no warning. The *British Medical Journal* carried a report on a twenty-nine-year-old woman who, after having been on the Pill for two weeks, suddenly collapsed. She was hospitalized immediately and died three days later. The autopsy revealed blood clots in two areas on opposite sides of the brain.

It started with a headache

In other cases there is a time of warning: the doctors call it a prodromal period. It may last for weeks or even months. The most common prodromal symptom is headache.

A tragedy that might possibly have been avoided occurred in Buffalo, New York, when Anne St. C., wife of a professor at a local university, mother of three and a user of the Pill, called her gynecologist and asked, "Is the Pill safe? Should I be taking it?"

Dr. K. snapped, "Of course it's all right for you to take the Pill. If it weren't, I'd never have prescribed it."

Anne did not tell the doctor the real reason why she was calling. In the preceding two weeks she had experienced several attacks of dizziness and double vision. She had also suffered from stiffness in the neck. If she had not been so readily cowed by the doctor's brusqueness, she might have detailed her symptoms. In that case, the doctor's reaction might have been quite different.

As it was, Anne had a stroke exactly eight days later. She was sitting at the dinner table and suddenly began to cough and choke. Her husband thought something had stuck in her throat and pounded her vigorously on the back. She continued to cough and choke. Their six-year-old cried out, "Look, Mommy's mouth is all twisted." Anne was partially paralyzed and totally unable to speak.

She spent two months in the hospital and then slowly recovered her speech and most of her physical functioning except for weakness in the right arm and leg.

A medical secretary in Houston, Texas, who had been taking the Pill for four years, had been having headaches for about a year. She blamed them on the fact that she was upset because her marriage was breaking up. As time went on, the pain became more severe.

The day of her stroke, she had washed her hair and put it up on big rollers. When she started getting a headache, she thought she had rolled up her hair too tightly. She was very tired and decided to go to bed. She noticed that her right arm and leg were numb and she felt "light-headed." When she got up to go to the bedroom, she walked haltingly. And once in bed, she slept very little because of the severe pain in her head.

On her way to work the next morning, she realized that she had suddenly lost the sight in one eye. In this case, a neurologist found a blood clot on the left side of her brain. She was hospitalized for a week. Her symptoms gradually disappeared. It took a month for vision to return and there is still a small blind spot after almost a year. She still has a slight numbness in her right hand. Her neurologist thinks that her stroke was caused by the Pill.

Another, more serious, case preceded by warning symptoms was reported in the *Lancet,* the British medical publication. The twenty-three-year-old patient had been taking the Pill for about six months. For about six weeks before she was taken to the hospital, she had been having attacks of double vision and for two weeks she had also had severe headaches. One morning she suddenly lost the ability to speak. Her left side was paralyzed. Twenty-four hours later she died. Autopsy showed the cause of death to be a blood clot on the brain.

Perhaps this patient's life would have been spared if she had stopped taking the Pill when she had her first attack of double vision. Drs. R. Thomas Bergeron and Ernest H. Wood of the Neurological Institute, Columbia-Presbyterian Medical Center, wrote in February, 1969: "The development of headache, visual symptoms or other signs of transient cerebrovascular insufficiency [meaning a temporary slowing down of the blood supply to the brain] should probably be interpreted as an indication for the immediate and permanent cessation of oral contraceptives." It can only be said that *perhaps* the above patient's life would have been saved, because Drs. Bergeron and Wood continue: "Even this is no guarantee that the clotting mechanism will return to normal."

Not all strokes are due to traveling blood clots. Some are due to hemorrhages of the blood vessels in the brain, and the Pill has been implicated in many deaths from this kind of stroke. The Royal College of General Practitioners in London has been conducting one of the largest and most highly regarded of the Pill studies. They found that the Pill was associated with this kind of stroke and that the association continued long after the Pill was discontinued. Both current and former users of the Pill were at greater risk from this kind of stroke than those who never used the Pill.

In Walnut Creek, California, these findings were confirmed at the Kaiser-Permanente Medical Center. Pill-takers stood more than six times the chance of developing hemorrhagic strokes than nonusers. There was also evidence that the risk of stroke increases with long-term use of the Pill. As with other circulatory and heart diseases, smoking, according to this study increased the risks posed by the Pill; the Pill and smoking together, multiply the risk factor.

Luckily, four people out of five survive their first stroke, although some are left like human vegetables; others suffer varying degrees of paralysis, blindness, speech difficulties, and other neurological impairment. Some victims recover completely because other parts of the brain are able to take over the functions of the area that died. This may happen spontaneously or only after lengthy rehabilitation.

There are also instances where the symptoms, such as numbness, light-headedness, or slurred speech, lasted no more than half an hour. Such episodes are believed to be caused by temporarily diminished blood flow to an area of the brain.

A typical such case was reported by Dr. J. C. Whyte of the Ottawa Civic Hospital in Ontario, Canada: "A 32-year-old woman who had been taking [an oral contraceptive] for two years experienced an episode of transient hemiparesis [weakness of one side of the body] and aphasia [inability to speak] which lasted 10 to 15 minutes. Following the attack, the patient underwent a complete neurological examination. There was no residual paralysis or other sign of neurological disease. An electroencephalograph (brain-wave test) recorded a few days later was normal. The contraceptive was discontinued and no further attacks occurred."

In other instances partial or total recovery is slow and comes only after a painstaking and usually expensive process of retraining and rehabilitation.

As early as 1969 the role of the Pill in CVA's suffered by young women was so well established in the minds of certain specialists—the neuroradiologists and neurologists who diagnose and treat CVA's in the living and the pathologists who diagnose them in the dead—that Drs. Bergeron and Wood wrote in the journal *Radiology:* "It would appear that there are now more than 100 well established cases of cerebrovascular complications associated with the use of oral contraceptives . . . [but] the number represents only a small fraction of the actual complications [because] physicians are becoming increasingly reluctant to report adverse reactions because of the risk of litigation."

Whether or not physicians report adverse reactions, there is an increase in litigation as more and more couples learn of the dangerous side effects of the Pill through tragic experience. Cary Ann and Bill P. are one couple among many who have sought redress in the courts.

Cary Ann married Bill when she was seventeen. Three days before her nineteenth birthday, she gave birth to a baby boy, Joel. A couple of months later, she went to a doctor for birth control help. He prescribed the Pill. Eight months after that, Cary Ann had a stroke. She was nineteen years old.

Cary Ann and Bill sued the drug company that manufactured the pill she had taken. The depositions, taken by the company lawyer, reveal in stark question-and-answer form just what a stroke can do to a young woman still in her teens. Cary Ann's lawyer, Mr. McD., stated at the beginning of the deposition-taking: "Mrs. P. will manifest, I believe, an obvious inability to answer a number of the questions you ask. We request that she be given time . . . and we offer to help answer the questions."

The record shows exactly what he meant. The drug company lawyer asked Cary Ann how long she had lived at her present address.

CARY ANN: I'm sorry, the numbers—

DEFENSE: Are you having difficulty with the dates?

CARY ANN: Yes.

DEFENSE: How old are you?

CARY ANN: [No response.]

DEFENSE: When were you born?

CARY ANN: I can't—numbers—because—ask him.

DEFENSE: Do you remember how heavy Joel was when he was born?

CARY ANN: Four and a—let's see, six pounds?

DEFENSE: Four pounds, six ounces?

CARY ANN: Yes.

Later on, the lawyer tried to establish just what had happened when Cary Ann had suffered her stroke.

DEFENSE: Were you with Mrs. P. when she had the episode?

BILL: No, we were over at her mother's. She went downtown shopping and came back and could hardly get into the door.

DEFENSE: Where did it happen?

CARY ANN: I was just walking back . . . I knew there was something wrong, but I didn't know what. I knew sometimes I was passing out—not passing out but—but—I don't know.

BILL: When she came in the door, her right foot was turned over sideways and she was dragging it. The right side of her jaw was coming out.

DEFENSE: What is the next thing you remember?

CARY ANN: I knew someone was there, but I didn't know what. I mean, my mother. I didn't know my mother. I knew Bill, but I couldn't—my son. I forgot that.

DEFENSE: After your stroke, did you have difficulty in walking?

CARY ANN: I couldn't walk a bit.

DEFENSE: How long a period did that last?

CARY ANN: Oh—

DEFENSE: Mr. P., did she have difficulty walking when she got out of [the hospital]?

BILL: I don't know how long it was before she got where she could walk again.

Cary Ann had lost the use of her right arm and hand and right leg for a while. Even after intensive therapy, they were still weak. She had had to have speech therapy, too, and still had trouble, as we have witnessed, in expressing herself. Cary Ann's lawyer then took over some of the questioning.

MR. MCD: Can you write your name?

CARY ANN: Sometimes, and sometimes I can't.

MR. MCD: Can you write anything else?

CARY ANN: Two or one.

MR. MCD: And numbers like you wrote for us today, you can write numbers?

CARY ANN: Yes, sometimes.

MR. MCD: Can you spell words? Could you spell "the" for me?

CARY ANN: No. You see, I can't—words like "the" and "it" and so forth. I could not—

MR. MCD: Can you lift your son? Are you strong enough to lift him?

CARY ANN: This hand, but not this one. Sometimes I can, just for a while.

MR. MCD: When you said this one, you meant your left hand?

CARY ANN: Yes.

Despite the physical and mental impairments caused by the stroke, Cary Ann, then twenty, had not lost one thing—her blond beauty. A quietly charming young woman, she showed an earnest desire to be responsive that so affected the drug company lawyer that he became misty-eyed and pulled out his handkerchief to wipe tears from his eyes.

Loss of speech

A neurologist in Washington, D.C., gives another reason for not reporting the Pill-linked strokes that he has diagnosed or treated. It has nothing to do with litigation. He says, "I assume that this problem is so well known that it doesn't need any further documentation from me. Every neurologist that I've spoken to has been very, very aware of this problem. It's been well documented in the medical literature for quite a long time." He added that he knows other neurologists who have treated twenty or more Pill-associated stroke cases that they did not report to the drug companies or to the Food and Drug Administration.

In the late winter of 1967, at the annual meeting of the Radiological Society of North America, Drs. Bergeron and Wood presented a paper that documented an increase in Pill-connected CVA's. They had studied the cases of all women in the twenty-to-forty-four age bracket who had been admitted to Neurological Institute in New York City in 1966 for cerebral angiography. This is a diagnostic procedure, a form of brain X ray, that is never undertaken lightly because it entails dangers. All the women in the study had suffered serious symptoms, such as unexplained loss of speech.

In some cases there had been no structural changes in the brain. In others the doctors were able to trace the symptoms to head injuries, tumors, or other "disease processes." In nine patients, eight of whom had been taking oral contraceptives, they found blood clots in the arteries of the brain.

The researchers then examined the hospital records for 1960, the year before the Pill was widely available to the general public as a contraceptive. There were only two cases of blood clots in the arteries of the brain in 1960 as compared to nine in 1966. One of the two was a patient who had just had a baby, and her case was considered "hormone-related."

In sum, Drs. Bergeron and Wood pointed out, there had been an eightfold increase in hormone-related strokes diagnosed at Neurological Institute in 1966 over 1960. The median age of the eight patients with Pill-linked clots in 1966 was thirty. Five were between twenty and thirty-four; three were between thirty-five and forty-four. The average duration of use of the Pill was sixteen months.

A thirty-four-year-old woman in the group, who had been on

the Pill for fifteen months, had complained of severe headaches. Suddenly her right arm and leg became paralyzed and she was unable to speak. Drs. Bergeron and Wood reported that both her mother and father had died of strokes. If this unfortunate woman's gynecologist had been aware of this background, then he apparently had not been aware of the fact that a family history of strokes should be a strong contraindication to the Pill.

"She was really very crippled"

In addition to strokes, the Pill has been associated with other cerebral disorders, including migraine headaches. Within a one-year period, Drs. Sherif S. Shafey and Peritz Scheinberg, neurologists at the University of Miami School of Medicine, reported on a group of thirty-four Pill users who all developed "neurologic syndromes."

In twenty-eight of these patients, the symptom was migraine. More than half had never suffered from it before taking the Pill. All twenty-eight lost their headaches when they stopped the Pill.*

The remaining six women had apparent strokes. Two made a good recovery. Two were left with disabling paralysis. One died. And the sixth suffered from a swelling of the brain, a condition known as pseudotumor cerebri (see below).

During the same period, one of the country's leading ophthalmologists, Dr. Frank Walsh of Johns Hopkins Hospital in Baltimore, became troubled about certain visual disturbances he and his colleagues were noting in Pill users. These disturb-

---

* Dr. Edwin R. Bickerstaff, at the Midland Centre for Neurosurgery and Neurology in Birmingham, England, told us that he had seen many patients with cerebral damage who developed migraine on the Pill and explained, "In true migraine many patients see flashing lights before their eyes and feel numbness or tingling in their extremities just before the headache and nausea set in. It seems significant to me that the young women who have been sent to me with cerebral damage often had preliminary episodes much like those of the classic migraine patient—even though they had not had a history of migraine."

ances were mainly of a type called neuro-ophthalmic: they are related to the nervous system behind the eye. In the *Archives of Ophthalmology*, Dr. Walsh discussed some of the patients who had come to his attention—including one who had died. He asked other ophthalmologists who saw evidence of a relationship between the Pill and eye disease to let him know about it. He asked that all reports be documented.

Within six months—with his associates Drs. David Clark and Robert Thompson—he had collected sixty-nine case histories that were published in the *Archives of Ophthalmology*. There was case after case of documented, disabling neuro-ophthalmic disorders.† This second study provoked enough concern among Pill-prescribing physicians so that, as Dr. Elizabeth Connell told the American College of Obstetricians and Gynecologists: "Many investigators have found themselves running an ophthalmology section in their contraceptive clinics."

Dr. Connell was just then reporting on a study that she and an ophthalmologist, Dr. Charles Kelman, were conducting together. They compared the eyes of Pill users with those of non–Pill users and found that the incidence of eye abnormalities in nonusers was far higher than they had anticipated. Most of the abnormalities "were actually not pathological in the sense that they produced visual damage" and not comparable to the disabling disorders reported by Dr. Walsh.

† Among the sixty-nine cases four were pseudotumor cerebri, suggesting the presence of a tumor. They are really due to benign swelling of the brain and, as Drs. J. P. Arbenz and P. Wormser of the University Eye Clinic in Zürich, Switzerland, have pointed out, could lead to an operation for a nonexistent brain tumor. Drs. Arbenz and Wormser had a thirty-eight-year-old patient who developed pseudotumor cerebri. She took the Pill for two months and then, because of nausea, switched to another brand. Within a matter of days, she became confused and had a severe headache and a variety of eye symptoms. Acting on hunch, the doctors decided merely to stop the Pill and keep her under close observation. If they were wrong, failure to hospitalize the woman could have meant death. Their hunch was right. The patient's headaches disappeared, and over the next few months there was slow but steady improvement of her eye symptoms. In Birmingham, Dr. Bickerstaff said he was seeing pseudotumors "in all sorts of young women, not just the classic type. Oddly enough, they're all on the Pill. And the symptoms go away when they go off the Pill."

"*Cataracts in both eyes*"

Many doctors breathed a sigh of relief at Dr. Connell's report, assuming that it had disproved or minimized the importance of Dr. Walsh's study. But Dr. Connell herself says, "Anyone who thinks *that* hasn't looked at my reports carefully. I have not disproved that the Pill may cause serious eye damage. . . ."

Eye specialists are also concerned about the possibility that the Pill may cause cataracts in humans as it does in animals, particularly since cortisone, a chemical cousin of the Pill, has been definitely linked to cataracts and other eye disorders.

A Detroit housewife wrote us: "About one year ago I noticed my eyesight was not what it used to be, and thought I needed stronger glasses. When I went to my optometrist to be examined he shocked me with the news that I had developed cataracts in both eyes. I am twenty-four years old and cataracts in someone this age are very unusual. I checked my ancestry to see if there were any cases of eye disorders or diabetes or anything that would contribute to this eye disorder. I even underwent various blood tests, and had a complete physical examination to determine what this was caused by, with no results. I was in perfect health except for my eyes. All the doctors I consulted suggested I should stop the Pill, since this seemed to be the only contributing factor. When I stopped the Pill, the cataracts progressed more slowly.

"It has been one year now that I have ceased to take the Pill. The cataracts are still there, of course, and the only thing that will rectify them is surgery, and even then I will have to wear very thick glasses to restore my sight."

Nobody knows exactly how the Pill causes strokes and neurologic or eye difficulties. Some researchers believe that rise of blood pressure may be a contributing factor. Other students of the Pill, such as Dr. William Spellacy of the University of Miami School of Medicine, have shown in biochemical studies that the Pill leads to an increase in large fat molecules that travel through the blood, piggyback fashion, on proteins and are associated with atherosclerosis (fatty deposits in the lining of the arteries). Still other concerned doctors point to the increase in blood coagulability as a likely contributing factor.

Many doctors are convinced that the Pill may cause serious and permanent eye disorders. One ophthalmologist we interviewed refuses even to hire an office assistant or nurse who is on the Pill. He doesn't want to relive the case of a thrombosed central retinal vein in a healthy young woman, his patient, Judy P., who had been on the Pill for five years and became permanently blind in her left eye. She was the victim of "thrombosis of the central retinal vein"—the vein had suddenly closed. "Although we couldn't prove it was the Pill, we couldn't prove it wasn't," her doctor said. "She was in perfect health. There didn't seem to be any other reason."

In a few cases, doctors themselves can inadvertently trigger extra precipitating factors that lead to strokes. Often, for instance, when women report disturbing symptoms, doctors advise them to switch to another brand of oral contraceptive; or they may prescribe a medication to alleviate the bothersome symptoms. A team of Swedish doctors reported an unhappy example of what can happen as a result.

The Pill and epilepsy

A thirty-five-year-old woman started on the Pill in May. In June she developed severe migraine headaches for which she was given ergotamine. The headaches returned periodically. In November she had a headache attack that was so distressing that she took five ergotamine tablets in a three-hour period. Then she became unconscious. Angiography revealed obstruction of the right carotid artery, one of the two major arteries supplying blood to the brain. An operation was performed, but she died soon afterward. At autopsy, a fresh clot of the carotid artery was found. Her doctors said they could not be certain to what extent the Pill alone might be held responsible for her death and to what extent her headache pills were a contributing factor.

It is now well recognized that women with a history of migraine and epilepsy make poor Pill candidates. The inserts packed with today's birth control pills warn that "your doctor will want to watch closely" these preexisting conditions. Many cautious doctors, however, simply will not prescribe the Pill for a woman with migraine or epilepsy.

There is even some suspicion that the Pill may cause epilepsy in rare instances. At least one housewife who developed epilepsy has received an out-of-court settlement from the manufacturer of the pill she had taken.

This New England patient took the Pill for more than three years and was carefully checked by her doctor. She suffered none of the usual side effects.

Then, like a bolt out of the blue, she had four epileptic seizures within twenty-four hours. The first happened while she was asleep, and her husband told her about it while they were having coffee. "He was telling me that I woke him up. The bed was shaking and my body was stiff and I was shaking.

"I just laughed it off and told him, 'You probably had a nightmare.' . . . I was just laughing at what I thought was my husband's dream when my right arm just became completely paralyzed." She was hospitalized, under treatment by her family doctor and a consulting neurologist. Oddly enough, she was taken off the Pill only when a drug company salesman—with whom her doctor had been discussing the case—disclosed that his company had a number of similar reports.

When this patient first developed epilepsy, she took four anti-convulsant pills a day. When we talked with her, she was up to ten. She says that she "has learned to live with it" and counts herself lucky that her husband's job is such that he can stay home mornings and help her. "I can't even take a shower without my husband being in the bathroom. So many things could happen."

Can anyone predict who might suffer a neurological catastrophe from the Pill?

Unfortunately, no. Many doctors today would not prescribe it for a woman with a history of migraine, epilepsy, or other neurological problems. But there are women like the twenty-three-year-old housewife who died in Germantown Hospital in Philadelphia and who had no history of such problems. Her case, reported in an April 1969 *Journal of the American Medical Association*, was the first recorded instance where both main arteries supplying blood to the brain were closed off by clots occurring within forty-eight hours. This is how Drs. Martin M. Mandel and William H. Strimel, Jr., of Germantown Hospital described the case:

"According to her husband, three weeks prior to hospitalization, she complained of 'numbness' of the left hand, which was characterized by a sensation of 'pins and needles in all of the fingers of the left hand.' There was no accompanying weakness, but later that day she noticed pain in both legs when walking. This was aggravated by bending as well as by doing household chores. On the following day, she had a 'urinary tract infection' and was seen by a local physician, who prescribed medication. This cleared up, and she remained well until two days prior to admission, at which time she had recurrent numbness of the left hand. Later that afternoon, the left leg and foot became weak and she complained of a generalized severe headache.

"On the following day, the weakness had progressed so that she had great difficulty in moving the right arm and leg. This was accompanied by slurred speech, with marked difficulty in expressing herself. She misused words and was soon unable to speak. On the day of admission to the hospital, she had become quite somnolent, and her husband noticed that she was unable to move the right leg. . . . Her husband related that she had been receiving birth-control pills . . . since the termination of her last pregnancy one year ago. There was no previous history of hypertension at any time. She had a normal pregnancy which was not complicated by hypertension or toxemia. Her parents are both living and well and there is no history of hypertension in either. . . . She died three days after admission. . . ."

At autopsy, Drs. Mandel and Strimel, Jr., found that although she was only twenty-three and had been in good health prior to this illness, this patient did have hidden arteriosclerosis (hardening of the arteries), apparently of long standing. The doctors concluded that the clot-producing factors of the Pill plus her already subtly damaged arteries were a deadly combination.

Another kind of neurologic case that Dr. Bickerstaff in Great Britain associates with the Pill is chorea, the uncontrolled twitching and jerking that used to be called St. Vitus's dance.

Five young women had been referred to him who had a mysterious chorea—not the kind that commonly follows rheumatic fever or pregnancy. Three had it so severely that they couldn't even do simple things like zip zippers or brush their teeth. And all five were on the Pill. As soon as he took them off the Pill, the affliction went away.

Dr. Bickerstaff said the onset is gradual. The patient notices that she feels clumsy, drops things, cannot thread a needle, fumbles at putting a key in a lock. If the condition does not progress beyond that point, she may never be referred to a neurologist. So his total of five Pill users who recovered from chorea when taken off the Pill may mean that there are many women with mild symptoms that are not noted medically.

Unless, as in so many other complications caused by the Pill, considerable damage is already done.

CHAPTER 6

Cancer and the Pill

In April 1969 Dr. John Rock, a co-developer of the Pill and professor emeritus of gynecology at Harvard University, agreed to answer questions about the Pill at a meeting of the Women's Auxiliary of the Massachusetts Medical Society. In response to worried questions, Dr. Rock assured the assembled doctors' wives that frightening stories about the Pill were "a pack of nonsense." When he was asked about women who had suffered adverse reactions, he replied, "It is clear that these women had case histories indicating that they never should have taken the Pill in the first place." For instance, Dr. Rock said, a woman whose family history is "replete with cases of cancer" is one who should not take the Pill.

As Dr. Rock well knew, scientists had first connected estrogen and cancer as long ago as 1896. By 1938, when Sir Charles Dodds in England synthesized DES—the first inexpensive estrogen product that was potent enough to take by mouth —hundreds of studies on the role of estrogen in carcinogenesis had already been published.

Within months of Sir Charles's discovery, synthetic estrogen went into widespread use as a treatment for women. Sir Charles was most unhappy about what he called the "promiscuous" applications of his brainchild. Indeed, it was not in England, where Sir Charles's cautionary voice was generally heeded, that the mass estrogenization of women first took place. Instead it was in the United States, and specifically at Harvard.

The first to publish on the benefits of estrogen as a "youth pill" was Dr. Fuller Albright, a leading scholar and researcher of his era. By the early 1940s many thousands of menopausal women were receiving DES, or similar estrogen compounds, which soon came on the market.

It seemed that the new DES was like Mount Everest. It was *there*, and scientists who like to tinker with female reproduction were determined to find a use for it.

Next after Dr. Albright, Dr. George Smith, of Harvard's gynecology department, got hooked on the notion that DES might strengthen pregnancies, prevent miscarriage, and even make "normal pregnancy more normal." Today it sounds bizarre, but Dr. Smith, along with his wife, Olive, a research scientist, gave thousands of women DES in the hopes of producing bigger and better babies.

Dr. Rock, a fertility specialist and a Roman Catholic, was interested in developing a hormonal contraceptive that would be acceptable to the Church. He knew that the estrogen treatments promoted by his colleagues, such as Albright and Smith, were highly controversial among cancer specialists. Rock's original hope for the Pill, which he worked on with Dr. Gregory Pincus of the Worcester Foundation, was that it might be an all-progestin product. (Progestin is a synthetic form of progesterone, the second ovarian hormone, and it does not at least have the same long-established connection with cancer that estrogen does.)

Rock and Pincus worked together during the 1950s. Their all-progestin compounds proved insufficiently effective, and so, regretfully at first, they added estrogen to the Pill. The possible link with cancer, at least in susceptible women, was, by his own admission, always in the back of Dr. Rock's mind.

Estrogen as a youth pill and a pregnancy treatment came into widespread use in this country in the 1940s. It was not until the 1970s—a time lag of more than thirty years—that a causal connection between these products and cancer was firmly established. In 1971 DES was shown to cause vaginal cancer in the daughters of women who had used it during pregnancy. In 1975 menopausal estrogens were shown to cause cancer of the womb.

The Pill was the last of these popular estrogen products to come on the market. It was approved as a contraceptive in 1960. Because there is such a long latency period in the development of most cancers, we may have no final answers on the Pill for a decade or more.

Meanwhile there are two schools of thought. Many scientists maintain that "estrogen is estrogen." All these compounds are metabolized in a similar fashion, and though there may be brand-name differences, what they are is most unclear. It is wishful thinking, say these conservatives, to expect that the Pill will be safer than DES or Premarin.

When Dr. Roald N. Grant, editor of *CA*, a journal published by the American Cancer Society, interviewed Dr. Roy Hertz at the National Institutes of Health, the following dialogue ensued:

DR. GRANT: Some physicians are apprehensive about the carcinogenic hazard of protracted use of steroid hormones. Is there any real basis for concern?

DR. HERTZ: Yes, there is. . . . For many years the profound effects of hormones on cancer of the breast and female genital tract have been known. . . . In addition, we know that estrogens, when given in large doses over a prolonged period, will induce tumors of the breast, cervix, endometrium, pituitary, testicles, kidney and bone marrow in mice, rats, rabbits, hamsters, and dogs.

DR. GRANT: Is there any reason to believe that the results of animal studies are applicable to man?

DR. HERTZ: Yes.

DR. GRANT: You believe that women who use steroid contraceptives for prolonged periods run a risk of eventually developing cancer?

DR. HERTZ: Yes. There is some risk, and the extent of the risk is undetermined. It is therefore mandatory that carefully designed studies be carried out to resolve this problem as quickly as possible.

Other scientists are more hopeful or perhaps more cavalier. They think that perhaps the progestins in the Pill may somehow cancel out the carcinogenic effects of the estrogen. Alas, this has not proved true in mice. In 1969 Dr. Thelma Dunn, a pathologist at the National Cancer Institute, reported at the annual meeting of the American Association for Cancer Research that she had solved the previously insurmountable problem of persuading animals to swallow birth control pills. She dissolved the Pill in liquid Metrecal and fed it to female mice. Four of the mice died immediately, and the remaining eight got cancer.

Breast cancer

Concerning the Pill and breast cancer, the jury is still out. Dr. Robert Hoover, Head of Environmental Studies at the National Cancer Institute, feels there is now considerable evidence that "estrogen per se" may be related to breast cancer in long-term users. As far as the Pill goes, the situation, he says, is "still muddy. . . . The most important questions have hardly been probed. . . . We don't know what the latent period is, we don't know how the Pill affects girls of sixteen differently from women of forty. We suspect that pre- and postmenopausal breast cancer may be two different diseases."

Two important but confusing studies were published late in 1979. Both implied that the risk factors are different for different groups. The first study, performed by Dr. Ralph Paffenbarger of Stanford University and published in the journal *Cancer*, indicates that women who have a history of benign breast disease and who take the Pill before the birth of their first child may substantially increase their breast cancer risk. Six or more years of use in *any woman* with a prior history of benign breast disease may also be an invitation to cancer—if Dr. Paffenbarger is correct.

Meanwhile, in England, Dr. Martin Vessey and Sir Richard Doll, both professors at Oxford University, compared 621 breast cancer patients with an equal number of controls. Their findings were published in the *British Medical Journal*. In forty-six-to-fifty-year-olds, women who had taken the Pill got more breast cancer, but in forty-to-forty-five-year-olds they got less. Curiously, women who had never used any contraception, not even the diaphragm or withdrawal, were the least likely to develop breast cancer, leading Dr. Vessey to speculate that perhaps infertile women with "less need" for contraception also have lower breast cancer risks.

Meanwhile, Dr. Hoover's hunch—an informed one, but only a hunch at this point in time—is that those most apt to get breast cancer from the Pill would (a) have had a family history of the illness, (b) have had a personal history of benign breast disease, and (c) have started the Pill at an early age.

Like Dr. Roy Hertz and many other researchers, Hoover is also concerned about tumors in other susceptible sites.

The liver and pituitary

Women who take the Pill for more than three years run a one-hundredfold increased risk of developing liver tumors, which are often fatal. Former Pill users may also be developing high rates of tumors of the pituitary gland. These seem most apt to occur in women whose menstruation does not return when they stop the Pill.

The ovaries

Long-term Pill use alters the ovary and gives it an abnormal appearance. Curiously, however, some studies—but not others—indicate that ovarian cancer may be *less* common in women who have used these hormones.

The uterus

How does the Pill affect the uterus? Thus far we know that it leads to an increased growth of benign fibroid tumors. These aren't fatal, but neither are they pleasant when they get out of hand. Hysterectomy is a frequent outcome.

Some Pill enthusiasts, such as Dr. R. T. Ravenholt of the Agency for International Development, remain hopeful that the Pill may prove protective against cancer of the uterus.

The life-styles game: the cervix and skin cancer

Almost from the beginning, doctors observed that the cervices of Pill users looked different. There was much controversy over what these changes signified. Dr. Louis Hellman, who was Chairman of the Food and Drug Administration's Advisory Committee on Obstetrics and Gynecology, made the enigmatic remark, "It's quite obvious that something is going on in the cervix, but what it is we don't know." One researcher, hematologist John Lindenbaum, demonstrated that some abnormal Pap smears in Pill users were linked to folic acid deficiency and could be reversed with vitamin supplements.

Beginning in the fall of 1965, Dr. Myron R. Melamed, a pathologist at Memorial Sloan-Kettering Cancer Center, performed a monumental study of 35,000 Pill users. Early cervical cancer was significantly more prevalent than in the diaphragm-using control group.

The study was so controversial that it could not be published in the United States. Finally, after long delays, it appeared in the *British Medical Journal.* Dr. Melamed lost his funding and was forced to abandon his Pill research. Subsequently, numerous other investigations confirmed what Melamed had found. Early cervical cancer—a condition that, luckily, has a very high rate of cure—occurs much more commonly in Pill users than in other women. Nine or 10 out of each 1,000 Pill users will develop cervical cancer according to current estimates.

Yet many scientists are reluctant to indict the Pill. They think that cervical cancer may be linked to a virus carried by the male. Pill users, they suggest, may have a greater range of sex partners. Also, the diaphragm, the condom, and perhaps spermicidal foams or jellies might offer protection or a barrier against the virus.

Most recently, a study has linked the Pill to malignant melanoma, a fatal skin cancer that used to be called the "black death." Further investigations are under way, but here again Pill "lobbyists" or apologists have introduced the "life-style" defense. Malignant melanoma is also known to be influenced by exposure to the sun. Pill users, the argument goes, may include a higher proportion of bikini-clad women who lie around on beaches.

Nonetheless, Dr. Hertz, with others, fears that in time the increase in cancer stemming from the Pill may reach staggering proportions. He points out that "the period of incubation of a cancer induced by a chemical carcinogen may be as long as twenty-five years."

Cancer-prone families

When a cancer-causing substance is applied to a strain of animals, the animals frequently have an all-or-nothing response. They all get cancer or none do. Among humans, some families appear to be much more cancer-prone than others. In 1967 a study of 1,802 breast cancer patients was reported in the *Annals of Surgery*, which described mammary cancer as a "familial disease" and pointed out that it appears to develop at a younger age in the women of each succeeding generation.

Surely, then, as even Dr. Rock, a father of the Pill, has cautioned, women from cancer-prone families might be prudent to avoid it.

The trouble is that twentieth-century birth control medicine is usually impersonal. Perhaps in the good old days, when most of us had family doctors, we could expect our doctor to remember that Aunt Millie died of breast cancer. Today's patient is well advised to keep her own record of her close relatives' major illnesses and causes of death. Today's patient should also be suspicious of any doctor or clinic that does not take a careful history.

A student who sought counsel at a center in New York City told us that when she tried to volunteer a few words about her family history, the interviewer responded firmly, "Look, this is no family history. It's just about you. I'm not interested in your family."

The young woman said, "But my grandmother died of diabetes. That means I'm susceptible to it. So how can you know whether the Pill is right for me?" The interviewer replied, "Well, my *mother* died of diabetes, but nobody in my family has it. So it doesn't mean a thing."

The patient persisted: "I've heard that the Pill can cause cancer. . . . One of my relatives had cancer. So maybe the Pill will give me cancer." She was told, "What happened to them will not necessarily happen to you."

Significantly, the Pill is the most popular birth control method prescribed at organized family planning clinics in the United States. Two thirds of the women who receive their contraceptive advice from these clinics use the Pill, a rate at least three times as high as that of women who go to private doctors. Clinic patients are also less likely to have thorough checkups, bringing out such subtle factors as elevated blood fats, which may increase cancer risks in Pill users, as well as the risks of cardiovascular disease.

A final word about estrogens as compared to other carcinogens: hardly a week passes that we do not hear of a newly discovered link between cancer and some substance in our environment. Perhaps it is tempting to give up, to stop caring, to shrug our shoulders and ride with the risks. Do bear in mind that many carcinogens are only "occasional." How many maraschino cherries, for example, does the average person eat? The Pill, like heavy smoking, is different, for it's a constant presence, a constant assault. Women who take the Pill are playing biochemical roulette with cancer, on a daily basis.

CHAPTER 7

Diabetes and the Pill

In a large percentage of the women who take the Pill, the body's ability to use the sugars in food is undermined. Many of these women develop prediabetic states, which show up as impaired glucose tolerance in laboratory tests. A few of them go on to develop overt, or clinical, diabetes.

Dr. John Tyson explained this phenomenon to us. "Growth hormone is increased in excess in Pill users. If you take an animal, any animal, including the human, and feed him growth hormone for seventy-two hours or ninety hours, you'll make him diabetic, because growth hormone antagonizes insulin and antagonizes the uptake of sugar."

Dr. Tyson studied two groups of women: five who were on the Pill, and five who had never taken it. The women both had identical glucose tolerance curves, but the women on the Pill ". . . put out five times more insulin to do the same job. God has given their pancreas the ability to do this. They take more insulin than the non–Pill users to do the same job. But just by looking at plasma glucose in lab tests, you would say everything is great.

"The girls who have abnormal glucose tolerance can't compensate by putting out more insulin. And these girls in my series are turning out to be the ones who are overweight."

Dr. Tyson is concerned about the relationship of overweight

and diabetes. After decades of study, we still don't know whether people become overweight because they are diabetic or diabetic because they are overweight. But we do know that anyone who gains a lot of weight often has a diabetic or prediabetic state, plus various other potentially life-threatening problems with fat metabolism, blood vessels, and nerves.

Dr. Tyson is apt to become rather vehement about overweight. "Because obesity and diabetes go hand in hand, [overweight women] are being subjected to a most unreasonable risk of diabetes. If anyone gains more than eight pounds on the Pill, I take her off."

If Dr. Tyson had been treating Jane G., he would have recommended stopping the Pill. Jane gained twenty pounds in the year and a half she took the Pill, "but I really liked it because I had been so skinny.

"Within eight weeks after I went off, I gained fifty pounds. I would stay away from sweets and still gain. I didn't have a period for almost two years. . . ." Jane is not the only Pill patient to find that weight gain is but one part of a complicated set of health problems they developed with the Pill.

Dr. Tyson, slim and attractive, was deeply perturbed by severely overweight women who stay on the Pill. "I've seen them," he says indignantly, "women who are 20 and 25 percent over their ideal weight. Big!—185 pounds! 205 pounds! They won't diet. And they won't use the IUD. And they won't have their tubes tied. And they can't be operated on because they are so fat. Do you know that as early as 1936 people were asking whether estrogens might be diabetes-producing?"

Apparently the drug companies haven't bothered much with that question. A recent ad for one of the birth control pills, aimed at physicians, features a full-page photo of an overweight, smiling black woman holding her packet of pills. "Give her the pill that's easy on you!" exclaims the headline.

But many concerned doctors have worried about estrogen and diabetes. And many of them don't like what they see.

Peggy D. took the Pill for about four years and suffered "terrific cramps" while she took it. Then she stopped the Pill to get pregnant. Now her daughter is six, but Peggy is still trying to regain her health. She suffered severe metabolic reactions, including a weight gain of almost seventy-five pounds.

"I went back on the birth control pills after the birth of our child, for about six months," she says, "because I spot-bled for three months." Then she stopped menstruating and now "I have a period about once a year. I'm depressed, want to cry all the time. No energy, I'm lifeless, uncontrolled some days. . . . I also have facial hair on my chin and neck; really, it's just a beard and mustache. I've lost all sexual desire. . . ." Peggy told us that she had her hormone levels tested and was told that there is nothing wrong with them. She is twenty-seven.

Peggy may be one of those women whose systems just over-react to the Pill. Researchers are beginning to look into a new and mysterious aspect of the Pill's effects. In most women who take oral contraceptives, the drug clears out of their blood rather rapidly, especially during the five days of the monthly cycle that require no medication. But in some women the Pill leaves a residue in the blood, which doctors call metabolites and which accumulate over time. These metabolites may explain some of the Pill's effects.

Researchers in many parts of the world have accumulated evidence linking the Pill to impaired sugar metabolism. Dr. Jack Goldman of Tel Aviv University Medical School told the sixth World Congress on Fertility and Sterility that his study of thirty-one women patients treated at Beilinson Medical Center in Tel Aviv showed the Pill to produce a significant change in glucose tolerance. Each of the women was given a glucose tolerance test before she started the Pill, another one after she had been on it for three months, and a third test three months after she had stopped the Pill. The second test indicated that the oral contraceptive had caused a "diabetogenic effect" in the women.

Fortunately, in the typical now-you-see-it-now-you-don't pattern of the Pill, the final test showed that their glucose tolerance had returned to normal after they discontinued the Pill. A control group of twenty-six women showed no change in glucose tolerance during the same period. Dr. Goldman concluded: "Diabetic women, or those with a tendency to diabetes, should either not be given this contraceptive drug or, at least, only with caution and under constant control."

It has been observed clinically that the Pill can make existing diabetes worse. The drug company literature now cautions: "A decrease in glucose tolerance has been observed in a significant percentage of patients on oral contraceptives. The mechanism of this decrease is obscure. For this reason, diabetic patients should be carefully observed while receiving the Pill."

Mrs. Glenda J., who is and was diabetic, was *not* carefully observed. She was put on the Pill in the days before its effects on sugar metabolism were generally known. In 1964 she went to her family doctor in her North Shore Chicago suburb and announced happily that she was getting married. She wanted to know if her diabetes would interfere with having a family. The doctor explained that he felt it was wiser not to plan on children. He advised her to take an oral contraceptive or an IUD. She preferred the Pill. He told her that she should get it from a gynecologist and recommended one. The gynecologist did not give Glenda an examination. When she called for an appointment, the nurse said that Glenda's family doctor had called and told them she wanted birth control pills. If she would come by the office, she could pick up the prescription.

Glenda was slightly nauseated at the beginning, even on her honeymoon. She was not concerned because she had heard her friends talk about this as a routine side effect of the Pill. She knew it was supposed to disappear after a while. The first few months of marriage were difficult. Not only did Glenda feel a little queasy most of the time, she also lost her interest in sex. Before they were married, she could hardly wait to be alone with her husband-to-be, Ken. But after they had been married for a while, things really weren't going the way she had hoped. She knew that it took time to "adjust." Her mother had warned her about that, but Glenda wondered whether her problem wasn't more than a problem of adjustment. She had simply lost interest in sex.

"They have no moral right"

After they had been married for six or seven months, Glenda began to have trouble with her eyes. She went to the eye doctor. He said that her problem looked like glaucoma to him—a frightening verdict. Her condition suddenly seemed to get out of control. She had a lot of pressure on her eye. As she described it, "It felt as if I were having little explosions." Her sight deteriorated rapidly. She was admitted to the local hospital. They recommended that she be transferred to one of the large hospitals in Chicago where there were many highly trained specialists. In Chicago the doctors recommended that she go to the Mayo Clinic. Her "glaucoma" was not really acting like glaucoma. And no one bothered to ask Glenda if she was taking the Pill. Finally, one doctor did. But it was too late by then. Glenda was totally blind.

Glenda was twenty-three when we learned of her case. She and Ken had built a "good life" together. Their house is spotless. Her aunt told us, "Glenda just has a determination about her. There's a will and there's a way. She gets down and washes the floors, for instance. She prepares all the meals and does her own housework. She baby-sits for her sister. She even changes the baby's diapers and everything." But Glenda will never be able to see her spotless house or her little niece.

Dr. William N. Spellacy was one of the pioneers in Pill research, and he studied its metabolic effects for several years at the University of Miami. That research proved that a significant number of women who took the Pill developed impaired sugar tolerance. The glucose tolerance tests for many of these women, when they were tested, appeared diabetic or prediabetic, although only a small percentage actually became diabetic. Dr. Spellacy, now at the University of Illinois in Chicago, has been studying the new low-estrogen pill for the past few years.

"It is significantly improved," he reports. "We're finding minimal changes in glucose tolerance. In many women we find no change at all." The new pills are far less dangerous, he believes, in terms of their effects on the production of growth hormone, the digestion of sugar, and the metabolism of fats. Problems in glucose tolerance are intimately related to other metabolic functions, including fat digestion, nerves, and changes in the blood vessels. "A woman going on the Pill today should ask for the low-dose pills," he advises. "I think 50 micrograms would be the highest to start."

When pills contain less than 50 micrograms of estrogen, "we'll see significantly fewer side effects" in sugar and fat metabolism, he believes. Since these pills have a higher incidence of breakthrough bleeding and certain other side effects, some women cannot tolerate them well. Some doctors still prefer to prescribe high-dose pills, as the breakthrough bleeding is a "nuisance" kind of symptom that provokes annoying phone calls from patients. One not atypical doctor told us, "Look, the low-dose pills may be safer in theory, but I just get too many complaints."

The full effects of a drop in estrogen dosage have not been evaluated. Most of the research done on the Pill involves those pills containing from 80 to 100 micrograms of estrogen, because those have been the most widely used.

In 1978, the last year for which figures are available, only about 19 percent of the birth control pills sold in the United States contained fewer than 50 micrograms of estrogen; another 55 percent contained 50 units, and about 26 percent still contained 80 to 100 micrograms.

Not all low-estrogen pills are alike. The other hormonal agent in oral contraceptives, progestin, a synthetic progesterone, causes some of the Pill's side effects. Despite a number of studies, no rule of thumb has been devised to measure which oral contraceptive is safest.

Dr. Victor Wynn, an English endocrinologist who heads the Simpson Laboratory for Metabolic Research at the University of London Medical School, has spent twenty years studying the metabolic processes of women who take the Pill. He knows as much about the ill effects of the Pill, and their causes, as anyone in Great Britain.

Dr. Wynn is not in favor of the Pill. "First of all," he told us, "there's a moral issue involved. Doctors who are not trained in endocrinology are making all sorts of pronouncements about the wonders of the Pill. They have no moral right to assure women that the Pill is 'perfectly safe,' because they don't know enough about the molecular biology involved."

At this point, he took us to look at a chart on the wall of one of his laboratories. It was a large—about two feet by three—map of the metabolic processes that operate in every cell of the body. It is so complex, Dr. Wynn said, "that no computer yet devised could chart the complexities or follow the variations that may result from interfering with the metabolic process."

We believed him. His chart was called "Biochemical Pathways," and that was the only thing we understood about it. Dr. Wynn comforted us by saying that the average physician would not understand much more. The chart did convey, in a most vivid manner, what a vast opportunity exists for disruptions when there is tinkering with anything as complex as hormones and enzymes.

"I see impairment in women on the Pill," Dr. Wynn told us. "Their glucose tolerance tests are abnormal. They secrete an abnormal amount of insulin. Their metabolism resembles that of frankly obese women—not the woman who's a few pounds overweight, but those who are really obese."

Dr. Wynn was convinced that there are far more women with Pill-linked prediabetic symptoms than most doctors dream of: "Say there are so-and-so million women on the Pill. How many of them do you think ever get a glucose tolerance test? We know from our work here that if you take a group of women over thirty-five who have been on the Pill for, say, seven years, 80 percent have abnormal glucose tolerance tests. With younger women, the percentage might be quite a bit lower, even as low as 15 percent. But they haven't taken the Pill as long."

No cell is unaffected

Dr. Wynn was scheduled to lecture on the effects of the Pill at the University of London Medical School and invited us to attend, along with his medical students. A woman's normal glucose tolerance is 600 units, he told the medical students. If you take a group of young women on the Pill for three months, their glucose tolerance tests average out to 750 units. If they stay on the Pill longer, 80 percent will show significant impairment of their glucose tolerance and 18 percent will have demonstrable "chemical diabetes."

"Chemical diabetes" is the precursor of the type of diabetes that develops in middle and old age. Some young women on the Pill, however, have developed this condition relatively early in life. This happens because the liver, when it is experiencing difficulty in metabolizing glucose, causes the pancreas to increase production of insulin. The pancreas may produce insulin until it, in effect, exhausts itself. Then the insulin production lessens. The glucose is not metabolized. And an affected woman begins to show signs of diabetes.

"The main difference between men and women—at least in their metabolism," Dr. Wynn told his students, "is that women tend to have a preponderance of small, closely packed molecules of lipoproteins [fats that piggyback into the blood on proteins], whereas men have larger molecules. The total cholesterol level in both men and women is about the same, but men have bulkier cells with more fats in them.

"The machinery of metabolism is beautifully complex and harmonious. It is easy enough to dominate it by introducing substances like the synthetic hormones in the Pill," he instructed his students. "But we have no idea of what risks we run by assuming control of such a delicate process. After all, there is no cell in the body that is not affected by oral contraceptives—nerve cells, skin cells, liver cells, blood cells."

Later, Dr. Wynn told us, "We will never know what harm

we've done by the widespread use of artificial hormones. It would take twenty years of testing thousands of women to find out. It's totally impractical. I've formed my own conclusions: I wouldn't take a drug that produced these effects."

CHAPTER 8

How the Pill Can Spoil Sex

One of the unkindest tricks that the Pill has played on some women has been to turn sex into a duty instead of a delight. This certainly happened contrary to all expectations, but it fits the pattern of our age. To many women it seems as if modern conveniences like dishwashers, floor waxers, washing machines —and the Pill—along with all the miracles that were supposed to set women free, have freed them only to achieve more performance.

Studies performed at the University of North Carolina School of Medicine in Chapel Hill, at the University of Lund in Sweden, and by the Council for the Investigation of Fertility Control in England have all confirmed that a decrease in sex drive is apparently far more common in Pill users than is an increase. Anywhere from 25 to 60 percent of Pill users (depending on the study) experience a noticeable loss of sex drive. Dr. Michael Grounds reported in the *Medical Journal of Australia* that loss of sex drive is the commonest reason for discontinuing the Pill in his country. Some women lose their ability to reach orgasm; others report that they reach it much less frequently and with considerable extra effort. They no longer find stimulus in their accustomed presex play and talk, or in the caresses and positions that used to arouse them. Today a nonorgasmic woman who consults a sex therapist is usually asked, "Are you taking the Pill?" before any therapy is attempted.

The quality of a woman's sex life, unlike that of a man's, does not seem to concern the drug companies or the (male) research establishment. During the Pill's early days, and the first decade or so of its widespread use, no serious research addressed this question. Women who reported changes in their sex drive often heard that old refrain: "It's all in your head." But the male sex drive is considered so important by the drug companies that it is always studied in conjunction with new male contraceptives, just as it is almost always mentioned in arguments against the condom.

When the Pill—an early form of Enovid—was tested on men in the 1950s, eight psychotic men at a Massachusetts state mental hospital were given 10 mg a day. The sex drive of the mental patients, in general, was not altered by Enovid. Their psychiatrists kept an eye on them, and they masturbated as much or as little as before.

But one of the eight was found, at the end of five and one-half months, to have shrunken testicles; his scrotum was "soft and babyish," the doctor reported. His side effects were viewed more seriously, it appears, than the unexplained *deaths* of three Puerto Rican women in the early experiments with the Pill.

Therefore, although the Pill did indeed sterilize these men, the fellow with the shrunken testicles put a damper on follow-up research.

From speak-outs and interviews with self-aware women we have discerned several reasons why the Pill may spoil sex. The most common term we hear is "anesthesia." In altering the normal hormone cycle and vaginal secretions, the Pill in some way often forces a woman to strain more to reach orgasm. Becky L., a thirty-two-year-old dentist, explained it like this:

"After I went into practice, my patients taught me a lot that I never learned in school. In school they tell you about side effects, but only things like hemorrhaging or severe infection. They don't tell you much about the nuisance problems that might be caused by drugs. Antibiotics give a lot of people rashes and indigestion, which, as a patient explained to me, can be modified by yogurt or acidophilus tablets. Pain-killers like codeine, tranquilizers like Valium, *and* hormones such as those in the Pill do *something* to quiet certain nerve endings so you just don't feel as much, either bad or good."

After reading a magazine article that mentioned only in passing that some women experience a loss of sex drive on the Pill, a twenty-five-year-old Pennsylvania attorney wrote us: "I have been on the Pill since my marriage three years ago and have had no side effects to speak of, except for a little nausea at the beginning. . . . My husband and I were both miserable because I could not have an orgasm. I had never heard before that the Pill could be responsible, but I decided to stop for a while and see. For four weeks there was no difference. (I suppose the hormones were clearing out of my body.) I was almost ready to start the Pill again when—pow! Now I know that I'm a 'normal woman' after all."

Sex became a "bore"

Another woman told us she began to think of sex as an "absolutely ridiculous bore" while she was on the Pill. Both she and her husband were relieved that she found sex to be fun again after she stopped the Pill. "It almost ruined our marriage," her husband said. "I knew she liked sex. I was sure she was getting it elsewhere."

A fashion coordinator for a Los Angeles department store who is a member of the League for Sexual Freedom gave up the Pill because, she complained, "It was getting so that I was sure that even an orgy wouldn't turn me on."

"I *like* sex. I always have," another, older woman told us. Her doctor had placed her on a regimen where she took the Pill —on and off—to control a medical condition. "During the cycles when I have to take the Pill," she said, "I can still have an orgasm sometimes, but I have to strain for it. Other times, I don't come at all, which, believe me, is very unusual in my case. Only when I discussed this with my doctor did he—and, mind you, this was only after looking it up—well, he admitted that it wasn't 'all in my mind.' He said it seemed to be pretty well established that the hormones in the Pill could decrease sexual enjoyment.

"Thanks to me, my doctor now warns patients who don't have to take the Pill for medical reasons that this is one side effect they should look out for."

One young woman, who had been married for three years and had a small child, reported exactly what happened to her when she was on the Pill: "I was absolutely sexually apathetic. I had no appetite for it at all. Like it was the most disgusting thing in the world to me! Many times I would go into the kitchen at night to take the Pill—I kept it in the cabinet over the sink—and I'd look and I'd think, 'Oh, my Lord, we have only two pills left and we haven't done it at all this month.' I'd take a pill and go jump into bed, just out of guilt. It went so far that—well, I have a very virile husband, but my whole attitude upset him so much that he was impotent several times. He simply could not get an erection. This was really a sad thing. Even when I stopped the Pill it took a long while for me to come back to the way I was before, a couple of months, really."

The next most common explanation of why the Pill can spoil sex for a woman is general ill health, on a minor scale. Caroline M. was quite typical. "My breasts were bloated and hypersensitive, so I couldn't enjoy the usual stimulation. I had leg cramps, so I couldn't get on top, which is my best position. Half the time I had a vaginal infection and an awful itch down there. The drugs they gave me for the vaginal infection made me constipated. I was very tired, and once I fell asleep in the middle of sex. When I went for blood tests they told me that I had a folic acid deficiency."

Caroline's vaginal infections are very common among Pill users. So is VD. The Pill, by interfering with the natural secretions of the vagina, leaves women susceptible to a variety of infections, including syphilis and gonorrhea. Those who use the Pill develop VD, other sexually transmitted infections, and vaginitis twice as often as the female population as a whole.

The Pill neutralizes normal vaginal acids, which protect

women against gonorrhea. It also increases vaginal carbohydrates, which encourage the growth of bacteria responsible for other infections. When Caroline switched from the Pill to the diaphragm, she took a big step toward protecting herself from a number of infections that range in seriousness from annoying to disastrous. The spermicide used with the diaphragm and cervical cap, as well as Delfen and Emko foams, provide some added protection by killing organisms that carry VD as well as herpes, trichomonas, and monilia infections.

If a woman who takes the Pill has relations with a gonorrhea-infected man, the chances are nine out of ten that she will also develop gonorrhea. With no contraception at all, the chances are only one out of three. With a condom, foam, or the diaphragm plus a spermicide, the chances that she will contract the disease drop considerably.

The third way the Pill spoils sex is through major illness. Women can get major health problems: Kitty G., for example, admitted, "If they ever leave me alone with the doctor who prescribed the Pill I will plunge a scissors in his heart and kill him. My stroke has left me semiparalyzed on my entire left side. My eyelid and my mouth droop. I cannot button buttons. I limp. I can't do sports anymore or stay in shape. I'm ugly. Everything takes twice as long as it should, and I'm a drag to my poor husband. I feel that he wants to leave me, but he's a moral person and he never will. For God's sake, how could a woman like me enjoy making love anymore?"

Finally—and this is more complex—the Pill can be a sledgehammer in the power balance between the sexes. Millions of women feel that they enjoy "it" less but must do "it" more. A study of coeds at a midwestern university revealed some dismal information. Those on the Pill had nightmares about bodily mutilation. They felt unable to say no to their boyfriends, but also believed themselves to be at a competitive disadvantage if they did not take the Pill. They were notably less orgasmic than the women who used other methods, but were less frightened of pregnancy and believed themselves more autonomous or in control. An editor at a news magazine, who is now thirty-five and "happy" but feels that she "barely survived" the social movements of the late 1960s and early '70s, explained, "I felt like an ever-ready sex battery. I had no excuse for saying no, no time to think. Month after month I got to loathe myself more. I think that the Pill and the other "instant" contraceptives like the IUD are the worst thing that ever happened to the female sex. Take away that tiny chance of pregnancy, that question of commitment or consideration, and what have you got? A woman is like those blown-up dolls which sailors use to masturbate."

Lisa G. also found the Pill's freedom costly. She is a political activist and often works at close quarters with men. During one assignment she spent long, isolated hours with Walter. They liked each other at once and found that they spent long periods just talking. Lisa found herself greatly attracted to Walter, and when he suggested they have sex, she felt there was no reason to say no.

Afterward, Lisa felt obliged to tell Timothy, her boyfriend, what had happened. They had always observed total honesty with each other.

"Timothy was utterly destroyed," Lisa explained soberly. "Our relationship was so beautiful. But after 'the episode' it was never the same. I blame myself completely. We dragged on together a couple of months more and then it was all over. He trusted me and I let him down. And it wouldn't have happened except for the Pill. When Walter sort of closed in sexually, I didn't seem to have any excuses. I know I should have resisted, Pill or not. I don't want to sound stupid about it. But I've given it a lot of thought. I can only stand myself if I give myself to one man at a time. And with the life I lead, there will be other temptations like Walter.

"I'm not on the Pill anymore," Lisa told us. "I'm going to get a diaphragm and keep it at home."

About half the women on the Pill report a neutral-to-positive effect on their sex lives. They appreciate the increased security, improved "aesthetics," and freedom from untimely interruptions. Many seem unaware that these benefits can also be achieved with methods that are harmless to women, such as the male vasectomy or the cervical cap (see Chapter 15).

For a few women the hormones in the Pill are overstimulating. They respond with what is technically called nymphomania, as recorded by psychiatrist Francis J. Kane at the University of North Carolina at Chapel Hill.

Dr. Kane told us about one young woman whose sex drive increased on the Pill to such an extent that she became terribly excited just by the act of walking. Her husband accommodated her by coming home for lunch so that they could have sex three times a day. But this was not enough. She wanted sex "all the time" and was most uncomfortable both physically and psychologically. "A nice girl doesn't feel this way," she told the doctor. She returned to normal as soon as she went off the Pill.

The reasons why the Pill so often spoils sex have not received definitive attention from scientists. A few have done some interesting work with monkeys that may or may not be applicable. Luckily, women are learning to trust their own experience, to analyze it, and sometimes to speak out. Based on the reports of users, the Pill may be a sex spoiler for several reasons, emotional, physiological, and even anatomical.

It isn't easy for women to describe their sexual feelings. Something in our culture and our upbringing inhibits us. Most of the time we take our cues from men, our lovers, or even our doctors and psychiatrists, and we merely parrot what they expect us to say. The author of this book has conducted many rap sessions on birth control, usually with women as the only participants. Once, however, in a church in Charleston, South Carolina, most of the women brought their lovers or husbands, leading to an unusual focus on the methods available to males.

One couple brought their baby as well. The father had agreed to tend to her, and did, carrying the infant in a contraption on his chest and soothing her when she got fretful. The mother felt impelled, perhaps in gratitude, to bring up a topic that was troubling her husband. "The condom," she said, "is like doing it with a raincoat or galoshes!"

Something in the way that she glanced at him for approval

led me to suspect that this wasn't her own idea. "Let's take a secret ballot of the women here," I suggested. "Write 'yes' if you know for sure when your lover is wearing a condom. . . . Write 'no' if the truth is that you really cannot tell."

There were twenty-eight women in the community room of that Charleston church. Twenty-eight ballots were received and opened by my daughter. To our astonishment, every one of the twenty-eight read "no."

Later, one of the women took us aside. "I've given this some further thought," she admitted. "Once in a while, if I'm not at all aroused and very dry inside, then I think I might find the condom an extra irritant. But when I *want* sex, when I'm lubricating, I can't feel its presence at all."

Some men find that "skin" condoms, or, indeed, any that are prelubricated, are much less objectionable than other brands they may have tried. In any case, since young men tend to ejaculate too quickly for the satisfaction of their partners, the slowing effects, if they exist, might actually be of benefit.

CHAPTER 9

Sterility and the Pill

For the better part of a decade, it was believed that women who stopped using the Pill, for whatever reason, became super-fertile. Doctors advised patients that if they did not wish to conceive immediately after they went off oral contraceptives, they should practice double contraception.* For example, some doctors recommended that the wife use foam *and* the husband a condom. In that way women could be sure to avoid what had become known as "the rebound effect" of the Pill.

Now doctors have become even more concerned about the Pill's ill effect in exactly the opposite direction: what they call "the oversuppression syndrome" or, in plain language, infertility. One distinguished physician to whom we talked considered this "the most tragic of all Pill side effects."

It is an established fact that a certain number of women simply do not start having their periods again after they stop taking the Pill. Others have irregular or scanty periods. In either case, they may find that they cannot conceive. They are sterile.

In the majority of women, post-Pill sterility is temporary and they will be able to conceive when their bodies return to nor-

---

* Many doctors now strongly advise their patients against planning to become pregnant until several months after they stop using the Pill and return to a normal hormonal equilibrium. This sensible advice would avert many miscarriages, although it is usually offered to protect the planned baby from the unknown effects of exposure to hormones.

mal. This process may take only a few months. The time lag can, however, be long: in a British study of post-Pill conceptions, the Pill users didn't catch up to the unmedicated group until forty-two months, on average, after they stopped taking the Pill. Three and a half years is a long time to wait to conceive a baby, long enough to make a joke of the phrase "family planning." Since many of today's women postpone their first child until they are in their early thirties, such a lag could subject them to high risks of bearing a deformed or retarded child, as well as significantly higher risks to their own health.

Some women pay a high price before their fertility returns. Joanna K. married at eighteen, and at twenty she became pregnant while taking the Pill. She miscarried, and was told that she had lost twins (twins are somewhat more frequent among women who conceive while on the Pill). Then "I miscarried three times with no explanations why. At twenty-two I was informed I would never have a child and that a hysterectomy was needed. . . ." Joanna didn't want a hysterectomy, she wanted a baby. After treatment by a fertility specialist, she conceived again, but lost this baby. Two other pregnancies also ended in miscarriages. Finally, after eight pregnancies, Joanna delivered a healthy child in 1977. She was twenty-six.

"My husband and I fought a lot during our struggle for a child," she says, "but now we are able to communicate easily and can understand the emotional changes which both of us went through before Mary Alice was born. I am scared of future miscarriages emotionally and I don't know why I had seven miscarriages after having been on the Pill for two and a half years."

Some doctors believe sterility is caused by such local injuries as damage to the ovaries or the lining of the uterus. These injuries, in turn, may be related to nutritional deficiencies caused by the Pill (see Chapter 14). Others suggest that the Pill may disrupt the functions of "hypothalamic cycling" or the pituitary gland, meaning that the centers in the brain that control ovulation have become sluggish or been knocked out of kilter by the Pill's artificial hormones. The greatest experts are the first to admit that they don't really know the cause of the problem. Britain's Sir Charles Dodds, Bt., M.V.O., F.R.S., the physician and biochemist who was the first to synthesize estrogen, said, "We should always be humbled when we think of what we do not know about the female reproductive cycle. We still have no understanding of the mechanism that makes one Graafian follicle in one of the ovaries of a normal woman maturate and ovulate each month. This is a baffling problem. Until we know that mechanism that selects one Graafian follicle, out of perhaps hundreds of thousands, to maturate each month, we still have to proceed with caution on any long-term, hormonal treatment of the human female."

Hormonal treatment need not even be long-term to trigger sterility. Dr. Miriam Furuhjelm of the Karolin Sjukhuset in Stockholm reported the case of a girl on the Pill who entered menopause at eighteen. "Most certainly, such a girl must be considered as seriously mutilated," Dr. Erik Ask-Upmark of the University of Uppsala commented.

Medical recognition of the "oversuppression syndrome" was slow. The first major alert was a report by Dr. M. James Whitelaw, a fertility expert, and his colleagues Drs. V. F. Nola and C. F. Kalman, which appeared in the *Journal of the American Medical Association* in February 1966. They described their findings with seventeen patients who had become infertile after using the Pill and seven who had become infertile after the injection of a contraceptive drug. Twenty-two of these twenty-four women had regular menstrual cycles before taking the birth control hormones. Only one was over thirty years old.

"Let's be honest"

One case reported by the Whitelaw group was a twenty-four-year-old woman who had had regular menstrual cycles since the age of twelve. When she married she used a diaphragm for a year. She stopped using it to become pregnant, conceived easily within a month, and delivered her baby normally. Then she took the Pill for eighteen months and stopped again when she and her husband wanted a second child. She failed to menstruate for eight months. Her gynecologist then referred her to Dr. Whitelaw. He performed a test known as a suction biopsy. It revealed that the lining of her uterus was badly damaged.

The report by Dr. Whitelaw and his associates challenged its medical readers with the words "Let's Be Honest About the Pill." To doctors, this phrase was recognizable as a jab at Dr. John Rock, one of the co-developers of the Pill and one of the men who had been disinclined to worry too much about its far-reaching present and potential dangers. Just nine months previously, Dr. Rock had written an article for the same journal entitled "Let's Be Honest About the Pill."

At the time, however, Dr. Whitelaw was a prophet without honor, at least to certain segments of the medical profession. The reaction to his article was immediate and electric. Doctors wrote scathing letters bitterly attacking Dr. Whitelaw as well as his conclusions. But the doctor had started an important ball rolling. Within a short time, many other physicians reported that they had been seeing the same symptoms in their own patients and began to report the histories of many more infertile women.

A little more than two months after publication of the Whitelaw report, Drs. H. L. Kotz and O. I. Dodek in Washington, D.C., noted: "Inquiry among colleagues leads to the conclusion that there are hundreds of unreported cases of protracted amenorrhea (no menstrual period) or marked menstrual irregularity and infertility following the discontinuation of the Pill." A year later, describing these case histories in greater detail in the *American Journal of Obstetrics and Gynecology*, these doctors reaffirmed the suggestion that "women should be cautioned about the possibility of . . . subsequent infertility before oral contraceptives are prescribed."

Apparently most young women who suffer from this "oversuppression syndrome" can be cured in time. At least their periods return, although not all can become pregnant. The required treatment is not pleasant. Often a woman must be admitted to the hospital for thorough investigation. Then she is usually treated with one of three potent drugs. One is a cortisone preparation with all its attendant risks. The second works through the pituitary gland. The third directly substitutes pituitary hormone and is still mostly used experimentally. The second and third drugs have been associated with multiple conceptions, not just of twins but, occasionally, of three, four, or more babies at once.

In other cases, nothing can ever be done for the patient, apparently because the Pill has destroyed the lining of her uterus.

In any event, the mental anguish associated with post-Pill sterility is incalculable. It takes many forms. Women who want to become mothers face the fear that they may have maimed themselves for life. There is guilt. There is anger at the doctor who prescribed the Pill. There is the anxious waiting. There is the costly medical treatment. There is tension that can turn every act of sex relations into a chore.

Mrs. Audrey K. told us that she had experienced every one of these reactions in the two years she had been off the Pill and trying to conceive. "I never, never had irregular periods," Audrey said. "I was normal and very heavy and never missed a period. While I was on the Pill, my periods were still regular, but after I went off, they became irregular and very scanty. I took a lot of tests, kept temperature charts and everything, and my doctor finally determined that my ovulation was abnormal, too.

"Finally, he sent me to a fertility expert. I go for treatment every two weeks. They check my tubes and my ovaries and do endometrial biopsies. Some of it's uncomfortable and the rest is simply godawful. The biopsy just smarts a little, but checking the tubes is bad. They shoot red dye into you and fluoroscope you and they do a lot of probing with instruments. It gets pretty painful. I have to stay in the hospital when they do it.

"It's made my husband feel terribly guilty," Audrey said worriedly. "At first, he kept saying, 'Impossible. The Pill couldn't have done it.' Now he feels just awful."

The most conservative approach to post-Pill sterility is apparently watchful waiting, but this requires endurance on the part of both patient and doctor.

Dr. R. Pinkney Rankin of Charlotte, North Carolina, reported in the *American Journal of Obstetrics and Gynecology* on a twenty-four-year-old patient with no children. She had taken one brand of the Pill for thirteen months and then switched to a second brand for the following eight months. Twenty-two months had elapsed since she went off the Pill, and her periods, which had been regular before she went on the Pill, had not yet returned.

A second patient was on the Pill for one year and did menstruate a month after she stopped using it. Then she menstruated infrequently for a number of months and then not at all. After seventeen months she began to menstruate spontaneously, conceived two months later, and now has a healthy baby.

Recent studies—from both England and the United States—confirm that in young women who menstruate sporadically, and whose fertility therefore may be precarious or "borderline" to start with, the Pill is especially likely to tip the balance.

Do young women know that the Pill may make them sterile? Does the typical Pill-prescribing gynecologist warn them about the danger of sterility? In far too many instances, the answer to these questions is "No."

We interviewed two young women at a Western college with high academic standing. Both of them were on the Pill.

Maureen S., a junior, is an anthropology major. Despite her outstanding academic performance (she works as a research assistant for the head of her department), her one ambition in life is to be "a good wife and a good mommy." She has no plans for a career although she intends to remain "alert, aware, and committed" after marriage. She takes the Pill and worries about it because one girl at her college died last term from a blood clot on the brain. The gossip around the school was that she had been on the Pill.

"I don't know for sure," Maureen told us, "but she probably was. Just about everyone around here is." "Everyone" also believed that the dead girl's blood clot had been caused by the

Pill. Maureen said she planned to stop the Pill, but not until she gets married. And she had no immediate plans for that.

Maureen considers herself to be too much of an intellectual to read any of the popular women's magazines that have warned about post-Pill infertility. At the time we talked to her she had not the slightest notion that her years on the Pill may forever destroy her dream of being a "good mommy."

Helen B., a senior at the same college, is a short, plump, freckled redhead who looks more like sixteen than her real age, which is twenty-one. She started taking the Pill in her freshman year. She has read some of the medical literature and understands what the Pill's long-term effects could be.

"I'm not willing to give up sex," she said. "And I'm not willing to take the risk of getting pregnant. I have no choice." Helen did try the diaphragm once—for one weekend. Perhaps she had been more concerned about the possible effects of the Pill than she had been willing to admit to us. "I went to a doctor and got fitted, then I spent the whole weekend scared to death. I was scared it wasn't in right. I was scared it wasn't safe enough. The whole weekend was rotten, so I went back on the Pill."

Helen's notion that she has no choice of contraceptives is disturbing to find in such an intelligent young woman. There was just no other choice that she was willing to consider. Convenience outweighed danger. When we asked her if she were not concerned about some of the other effects of the Pill—all easily avoidable by switching to another contraceptive—she replied casually, "Every time you walk across the street you take a chance. I'm not going to stop crossing streets—or taking the Pill."

A personal reminiscence by Sir Charles Dodds is relevant to these students' situation. This is how the eminent British doctor told the story to a medical audience: "I used to be taken as a boy by a wealthy uncle to a resplendent seaside hotel which had the characteristic Palm Court orchestra. This used to produce saccharine music during afternoon tea, and I remember on one occasion my uncle and I arrived late and we had to sit next to the orchestra. I was astonished to hear a violent quarrel being carried on in undertones between the musicians. While *sotto voce* curses and imprecations were being bandied about, soft music was coming forth for the audience who had no idea what was going on beneath the surface. It may well be that this situation is similar to what is happening in the body [with the Pill].

"Just as the horrors of carcinoma of the lung have no effect on young cigarette smokers," Sir Charles concluded, "the vague potentialities of later years have no effect on young oral contraceptive users."

CHAPTER 10

Genetic Changes and the Pill

The threat of genetic damage is our number one health problem.

Damage sown in the germ plasm is far more dangerous to the human race than immediate clinical complications like cancer or thalidomide, which cripple or kill a single person, but are not reproduced.

The first of these foreboding statements comes from Dr. Marvin Legator, a biochemical geneticist. The second warning was issued by Dr. Cecil B. Jacobson, an obstetrician-cytogeneticist. They are two of the founding fathers of a new science called mutagenetics, whose cadre includes clinicians, medical geneticists, biochemists, molecular biologists, cytogeneticists, and experts in population genetics.

These men fear that a "genetic emergency" or even a "genetic disaster" lurks somewhere in the future of humankind. They are worried because more and more of the food we eat, the clothes we wear, the air we breathe, and the medications we take contain chemicals that may cause damage to an existing human fetus or—something they fear far more—cause basic changes (mutations) in the human genes (germ plasm) that might not be observed for a century or more after the first mischief was committed.

It will require future generations of mutageneticists to determine whether or not a pill taken today will also affect children in generations yet to come. Others are concerned about the more immediate—but still long-range—effects of the powerful agents, like the Pill, that we ingest. DES, the estrogen used to prevent miscarriages, produced heartbreaking side effects in the daughters who were so precariously carried. Some of these children, at or shortly after puberty, developed cancers and other disorders of the female organs; many of these had hysterectomies in their teens and early twenties, and some died. Nor did DES sons escape damage: they show an increased incidence of genital abnormalities, including cysts of the epididymis (part of the sperm transport mechanism), which may impair fertility, undescended testicles, and microcephalic penises.

Now it appears that the women who took DES may themselves be subject to higher than normal risks of breast and other hormone-dependent cancers. The DES Task Force of the Department of Health and Human Services recommends that these women avoid any estrogen drugs (such as those given for menopause symptoms and to suppress breast milk after birth, as well as oral contraceptives). Many members of the Task Force, including this author, also feel that women who were exposed to DES in the womb should avoid the Pill, a conclusion that seems only prudent.

The DES horror story raised a frightening question about the Pill: would children conceived while their mothers took the Pill show DES-type effects? Would the Pill affect children conceived within the first month or two after the Pill was stopped?

To date, there are no answers to these questions. A number of doctors we contacted reported that they had not seen any cases of DES-type symptoms related to the Pill. No one, however, is to our knowledge systematically tracking Pill babies as they reach puberty. In Washington, D.C., the Department of Child Health and Human Development is planning a study.

Women who have had babies exposed to the Pill, or conceived shortly after taking it, should inform their children and their children's doctors of the exposure. It might be particularly advisable to inform the doctor who cares for the child at puberty or the daughter's first gynecologist.

In light of what is known about DES, it is also prudent to ignore the drug manufacturers' instructions about taking the Pill for another month if a period is skipped. We feel that a woman should stop taking the Pill immediately if there is any chance at all that she is pregnant.

Condoms, diaphragms, and foam will probably not harm a developing fetus, but the Pill might.

Dr. David Carr of McMaster University in Canada found a striking increase in a rare chromosomal defect known as triploidy among the babies of women who conceive within six months after going off the Pill. Most of the babies with this defect die in the womb or at birth.

More miscarriages

Moreover, Dr. William Peterson discovered a significant increase in miscarriages and abnormalities in babies in a group of women who had used the Pill prior to becoming pregnant. Dr. Peterson, then the chief gynecologist of the U. S. Air Force, studied 1,141 maternity patients in the Malcolm Grow Hospital at Andrews Air Force Base in Washington, D.C. He separated previous Pill users—422 women—from non–Pill users.

The overall rate of miscarriage in former Pill users seemed reassuring. It was only very slightly higher than the incidence in non–Pill users, 9.2 percent as compared to 8.6 percent. However, when the doctor took into consideration the length of time during which the women had taken the Pill, and how soon conception had taken place after it was discontinued, the picture shifted. Women who had taken the Pill for two years or longer, and then conceived within one month after stopping the medication, experienced the dramatic miscarriage rate of 20 percent, or one in five. The incidence of major abnormalities among babies who had been conceived in the first month after their mothers had stopped taking the Pill was also strikingly higher than the number of defects in babies born to women who had not used the Pill.

Dr. Peterson concluded: "It may be prudent to warn those intending to conceive following use of the Pill to avoid pregnancy in the first month." Other doctors suggested deferring pregnancy for as long as six months after stopping the Pill. They point to findings that Pill users become deficient in certain vitamins and minerals. Among these are several of the B complex group (including folic acid), zinc, and magnesium. Common sense indicates the wisdom of giving the body a rest and a chance to return to normal after using the Pill and before trying to conceive.

It has now been proven that the Pill causes a deficiency of folic acid, which is considered essential for a normal pregnancy because it promotes growth and helps develop healthy red cells. Several groups of researchers established that women on the Pill have a lower serum folate level (see Chapter 14).

Tests with animals suggest that the effect of the Pill on the ovaries is a tendency for overripe eggs to become fertilized when the Pill is stopped. This may be responsible for some of the increased numbers of miscarriages and fetal abnormalities.

And no one as yet has established what processes may be triggered in a woman who becomes pregnant while taking the Pill (it happens more often than most people realize) and then, unaware that she is pregnant, continues to take it.

Women who take hormones during pregnancy, either as oral contraceptives or as morning-after pills, have a 25 percent greater chance of delivering babies with major birth defects and a 33 percent increase in minor birth defects, according to a study conducted at the Hadassah Medical School in Israel.

Children inadvertently exposed to synthetic hormones in the womb are especially likely to be born with defective limbs. Dr. Dwight Janerich of New York State's Cancer Control Bureau, testifying before the U. S. Senate in 1976, described a study which showed that such infants were five times as likely to suffer from defective limbs—missing parts of arms or legs—than infants who had not been exposed.

Cynthia A. conceived while taking the Pill. Her son "was born missing the little finger on his left hand, several bones in his left wrist, and his left forearm was short and shaped differently from his right. He was hyperactive and was diagnosed as a borderline learning-disabled child after extensive testing in elementary school. . . ." Peter is now in high school but just recently developed another bone disease of his afflicted arm.

Cynthia contacted us because she wants to make other women aware of "the terrible chance" they are taking when they use the Pill. About her son Cynthia suffers guilt, anger, and remorse. "I hurt for him every day, that I unknowingly caused him this condition," she says.

Some researchers have suggested that exposure to synthetic hormones may also affect a child's IQ. Psychologist Jean Jofen of New York City's Baruch College found that the children of the female survivors of Auschwitz had subnormal IQ scores in nursery school. Years earlier, their mothers had been subjected to the horrors of a Nazi concentration camp; one of those horrors was the administration of estrogen, which was added to their soup. The Nazis hoped that the estrogen would keep their female prisoners from menstruating. It did. But were the reduced IQ scores a bizarre side effect years later?

Tentative affirmation for this suspicion came from a research group in Puerto Rico. Younger children in Puerto Rican families generally have higher IQ's than their older siblings. When their mothers take the Pill to space births, however, the younger children do not show the same scores. They are still as bright as, or brighter than, their siblings, but the differences are less marked.

Some of the hormones in the Pill find their way into mothers' milk. Because the long-range effects of these hormones have not yet been determined and cannot be gauged until the first generation of "Pill babies" reaches adulthood, and perhaps not even then, a growing number of physicians have become adamantly opposed to giving the Pill to nursing mothers. Many flatly counsel nursing mothers against taking the Pill.

When doctors clash

Dr. George Thosteson, author of a widely syndicated medical column for newspapers, also objects to giving the Pill to nursing mothers. In one of his articles he pointed out that the Pill can result in a reduced flow of milk and suggested that his readers refrain from taking chances. He further suggested that the estrogens in the Pill, when transmitted to the infant through the mother's milk, might have a feminizing effect on a boy baby. Dr. Thosteson received a barrage of letters from worried women who had nursed their babies while using the Pill, but he stuck to his guns and wrote a second column on the subject.

Clashes between gynecologists and pediatricians over this matter have been occurring more and more frequently. Mrs. Francine P., for example, was breast-feeding her baby daughter, Katy. At her six-week checkup, Francine's gynecologist put her back on the Pill, explaining, "Some nursing mothers find that their milk supply diminishes when they take oral contraceptives. So if you run into any trouble, call me." Francine's milk supply was not affected and she continued to nurse Katy.

At her baby's three-month checkup with the pediatrician, *that* doctor asked Francine, "How is your milk supply? Do you need a supplemental formula?"

"No," Francine said and explained proudly, "I've been back on birth control pills for six weeks and it hasn't dried up my milk at all."

The pediatrician turned purple. She telephoned Francine's gynecologist and asked him angrily, in Francine's presence, "Don't you ever read a medical journal? Don't you know the hormones in oral contraceptives get into the milk? Don't you know that the long-range effect on the infant has not been determined? Don't you know that in some species of animals, when hormones are given to infants it makes them sterile? We don't even know if human beings are one such species! We can't know until the first generation of Pill babies grows up. Giving the Pill to a nursing mother is monstrous! You may be Francine's doctor, but I am Katy's doctor! On Katy's behalf, I am ordering Francine to stop oral contraception at once!"

While practicing physicians were thus embroiled, scientific investigation into genetic effects of the Pill was continuing. At St. John's University on Long Island, for instance, Sister Elvera Abbatiello was exploring the effects of oral contraceptives on the embryonic development of mice. Her findings suggested that when certain compounds are administered early in pregnancy, the temperament of the offspring may be affected. The males were calm and seemed to lack aggression. The females were more aggressive than normal.

The truth is that human knowledge about the effect of the Pill on genes had not progressed much since November 1966, when an article by Dr. Roy Hertz and Dr. John C. Bailar III appeared in the *Journal of the American Medical Association* summarizing what was then known. They wrote: "An unequivocal abnormality produced by estrogen-progestogen combinations is the suppression of ovulation itself. It is only reasonable to consider the ultimate fate of the ovum that would have been normally released from the ovary. We do not know whether this ovum dies or survives. If it survives, is it altered in any way? . . . the delayed clinical manifestations of many congenital abnormalities require that these children be followed for six to nine years in order to completely appraise any possible effects on them."

CHAPTER 11

The Pill and Jaundice, Thyroid Function, Weight Gain, Urinary Infections, Arthritis, Skin and Gum Problems, Etc.

Many doctors used to scoff at women who asked them whether this or that ailment could be caused by the Pill. The stock reply, not always put so bluntly, was, "It's all in your head."

The doctors scoff no longer. It is now recognized that the hormones in the Pill affect virtually every system of the body and may produce extremely bizarre responses. Dr. Louis Hellman, for instance, reported that when a patient asked him whether the Pill might be responsible for an increase in dandruff that had been worrying her, he had to tell her that he did not really know.

More than one hundred different side effects have been attributed to the Pill, and none of them are as "minor" as dandruff. Because it affects every cell in the body, the Pill can spread its mischief to unexpected organs. When the damage shows up in the liver, thyroid, gallbladder, or urinary tract, the results can be dangerous as well as painful.

The most recent disorder to be linked to the Pill is hepatitis, a debilitating and extremely dangerous inflammation of the liver. In Boston, the Collaborative Drug Surveillance program found that women on the Pill were over three times as likely to be hospitalized with acute hepatitis as other women. Public health doctors are still questioning this study, and many of them believe that some of these "hepatitis" cases were actually cases of Pill-induced jaundice that were misdiagnosed.

Jaundice itself is quite common among Pill-takers. The Pill apparently causes a woman's bile to get thick, and in some women it gets thick enough to block the small bile passages in the liver. The insert that is supposed to be packed with the Pill now warns that any woman who notices a yellowing of her skin should call the doctor immediately.

Pill jaundice afflicts young women as often as their older sisters, and women who develop it usually do so within their first few months on the Pill. Most cases clear up when the Pill is stopped. In 140 cases of jaundice reported in a three-year period to the Swedish Committee on Adverse Reactions, for example, 70 occurred within the first six weeks of Pill use, and most of the rest within three months. Half of the jaundice patients were under twenty-five. And, even though most of the 140 cases were considered "mild," 130 of the women had to be hospitalized for anywhere from two to ninety-five days.

Swedish researchers, as well as investigators in the United States and Great Britain, found that women who developed jaundice during pregnancy displayed a marked tendency to get it again if they subsequently went on the Pill. Preliminary results of a study of mothers, sisters, daughters, and other female relatives of women who developed jaundice after taking the Pill seem to indicate that certain families are predisposed to this ailment, and that these women tend to develop it during pregnancy or while on the Pill. Fortunately, most cases disappear with the end of pregnancy or when the woman goes off the Pill.

Jaundice also appears, however, in women with no family history indicating predisposition. Drs. Ulf Larsson-Cohn and Unne Stenram of the University of Uppsala reported one such case in the *Journal of the American Medical Association.*

The Swedish doctors wrote about a twenty-eight-year-old patient: "No previous hepatic [liver] or other serious illness and no contacts with jaundiced persons were known. She had never been pregnant. . . . After about two weeks [on an oral contraceptive] she experienced considerable itching and observed that her feces were gray." She visited the outpatient clinic of Akademiska Sjukhuset because of increased itching.

The examining doctors found that she was mildly jaundiced but had no fever. Her general condition was good. Yet four days later she was admitted to the hospital and a biopsy showed liver cell damage. She was taken off the Pill. The itching disappeared in less than a week, and the doctors reported: "She felt quite well when she left the hospital," a week later.

Decreased liver function

Another Swedish researcher, Dr. Anders Westgren, studied 134 women who had had no previous history of liver disease of any kind. After a year on the Pill, one sixth of these women showed pathological results. "There is a clinically significant decrease of the liver function caused by oral contraceptives without the shadow of a doubt," Dr. Westgren reported, "but these cases are relatively rare."

Drs. Robert K. Ockner and Charles S. Davidson, both affiliated with Harvard University, pointed out that "the case histories display a remarkable similarity. . . . After taking oral contraceptives for two weeks to several months (most often for four weeks or less), the subject may notice the onset. . . . Cessation of contraceptive therapy usually results in a complete clinical and chemical remission within a few weeks to a few months."

Dr. Howard E. Ticktin, associate professor of medicine at the George Washington University School of Medicine, reported that "liver function abnormality occurs in approximately 20 percent of women taking oral contraceptives." He finds, along with Drs. Ockner and Davidson, that the "changes are usually moderate . . . and are readily reversible upon withdrawal of the drug."

Some women will go to surprising lengths to see whether they can escape from liver symptoms. The *Medical Journal of Australia* reported the case of a twenty-three-year-old woman who developed jaundice a few weeks after starting on the Pill. Tests soon indicated that she had acute hepatitis, which cleared up several weeks after the Pill was stopped. When she resumed the Pill, she again became jaundiced. Again the Pill was stopped. Again she became well. Eighteen months later she again wanted to go back on the Pill, and did. Ten days later she was again struck by jaundice. Again she became well and again she returned to the Pill. One week later, her liver function was abnormal once again. Only at that point did this patient say farewell to the Pill for good.

The Pill also has serious adverse effects on the gallbladder, and women who take the Pill face an increased risk of someday facing surgery for gallstones.

Pill use causes higher levels of cholesterol saturation in the bile, according to a study reported in the *New England Journal of Medicine* in 1976. This high level of fat in the bile is considered "an early chemical stage of gallstone disease," according to Dr. Donald Small of the Boston University School of Medicine. Many of the women with this problem later form stones.

The risk of gallbladder disease rises with the length of time a woman has been on the Pill. It becomes marked after about a year and doubles in four to five years. In some studies, Pill users are two and a half times as likely to suffer from gallstones as comparable women.

One doctor who has long been concerned with the Pill's effect on the thyroid has concluded that all women show changes in thyroid function tests when they are on the Pill. This researcher, Dr. D. Winikoff of Melbourne, Australia, says that no one really knows what this means, but one proven consequence is that when such changes occur, they make it nearly impossible to diagnose thyroid disorders. Dr. Winikoff and other physicians advise that a woman must be off the Pill for at least two months before a doctor even attempts to obtain an accurate reading of her thyroid function. Other researchers have noted actual physical changes in the thyroid gland of Pill users.

Many of the symptoms that Pill users complain of—

chilliness, weight gain or loss, appetite changes, hoarseness, decreased sex drive, water retention, nervousness—are also symptoms of thyroid disturbance. Whether or not these symptoms in Pill users are linked to thyroid problems remains to be discovered. Also, after some women stop the Pill, they continue to have menstrual disturbances or water retention problems or to suffer from fatigue for a year or longer. It has been speculated that changes in thyroid functioning may be linked to this Pill backlash, but no conclusive evidence has been developed.

Mrs. Frieda Y. is typical of women who have experienced such problems. She used to be in pharmaceutical advertising. "I was a true believer in the Pill," she told us. "I knew it could affect some women badly, but I believed that the percentage was tiny. Besides I had always been healthy.

"At first I felt fine on the Pill, but then I began to suffer more and more from cold weather and I developed increasingly severe cramps and weakness for a week or so before my periods. I never associated this with the Pill. All the time I was still writing copy about how great it was. I guess I brainwashed myself."

"I felt ninety years old"

"But then it reached the point where I felt ninety years old before my periods and I couldn't walk upstairs. I was staying home from work a lot. My boss, who was an expert on drugs, noticed that there was a cyclical pattern to my attacks of weakness and suggested it might be from the Pill. I asked my doctor about it, and he said to stop and see.

"I've been off the Pill for a year and I no longer get sick enough to have to miss work. But I still feel like an old lady before my periods and I still have trouble with stairs. I still get puffy from water retention, although not as much as I used to. And I still get cold."

Since the Pill can cause distortion of the tubes from the kidneys to the bladder, thus interfering with the flow of urine, it also makes some women more susceptible to kidney and bladder infections. Researchers at the Welsh National School of Medicine in Cardiff screened 3,578 women for certain bacteria in the urine that are thought to represent an early stage of urinary tract infection. They found that "oral contraceptives were taken more frequently by the bacteriuric subjects [women showing significant bacteria] than by the controls"—that is, women who had no such bacteria. The researchers wrote: "Since many oral contraceptives contain estrogens, interference with the dynamics of urine flow may account for the higher prevalence of bacteriuria in subjects taking these drugs." In most cases, urine flow returns to normal within six months to a year after the Pill is discontinued.

Greta B. has been taking the Pill for five years. Although she has suffered from recurring infections for most of that time, neither she nor her doctor associated the infections with the Pill. "Ever since I've been married," she says, "I've suffered chronic bladder infections and get herpes at least once a year. My herpes covers my gums, my tongue, and around my lips."

Greta has had many X rays and has been treated with several different antibiotics. It is becoming increasingly difficult to manage her infections, since she has developed immunities to at least three drugs. "All the doctors can tell me is to wear cotton underwear and avoid coffee, Coke, and tea. . . ."

Before the doctors will be more helpful, they want Greta to undergo an uncomfortable and expensive series of tests. She has decided to give up the Pill and follow a good diet, supplemented by vitamins, to recover from her years with the Pill (see Chapter 14). We believe that she will recover, and hope that she can avoid further tests and drugs.

In addition to the changes made in the urinary tubes, the nutritional problems caused by the Pill may leave many women susceptible to infections. Pill users, for example, are far more likely to get chicken pox than other women. The risk of getting chicken pox or another herpes infection may be related to the deficiency of many vitamins, particularly the B vitamins, caused by the Pill.

Caroline J., a New Jersey college student, had been on the

Pill for six months when she developed cystitis, an inflammation of the bladder. She suffered from blood in the urine and frequent urination. Although Caroline had the best care of a well-known urologist, the disease continued to appear cyclically for the next year, every three months.

The second serious appearance of cystitis, the following summer, was accompanied by a rash that extended from Caroline's legs up to her chest. It was fiercely itching.

In addition, according to Caroline: "I began to notice the more common reactions to the Pill. I had gradually gained more than ten pounds, I felt bloated and sluggish and I was nauseated. Also, I had pains in my lungs and I was short of breath. The doctor said it was vein pains," possibly the first signs of an impending blood clot.

By the end of the summer, Caroline had had it. "I had been reading articles that tended to confirm the suspicions that I had had for more than a year. At the end of August I just stopped taking the Pill.

"I didn't realize how bad I had felt until I stopped. In general, I felt better immediately, and the vein pains disappeared within two or three weeks. Within a month and a half the weight gain was lost without dieting. Even my boyfriend felt better, since he had been worried about my feeling so bad."

What about the cystitis?

"Oh, it came again once, early in the fall, soon after I had stopped. I've never had it since."

What about the rashes?

"Gone, too, immediately. I am using a cervical cap now, and we both feel better about it. I'm convinced it was the Pill."

Drs. Giles G. Bole, Jr., Mitchell H. Friedlaender, and C. Kent Smith of the Rackham Arthritis Research Unit at the University of Michigan reported on eight women, all in their twenties, who either developed arthritis-like symptoms or, if the symptoms existed before they went on the Pill, found that the symptoms became worse. When the Pill was stopped, the symptoms stopped or got better. The doctors continued their studies and subsequently established the same pattern in another group of young Pill users.

The report prompted a letter in the British medical journal *Lancet* from Drs. Harry Spiera and Charles M. Plotz of New York. These doctors said: "Over the past three years we have seen 22 young women who . . . after beginning oral contraceptives developed [arthritic symptoms]. The joint swelling was usually limited to the hands. On cessation of the oral contraceptive, the symptoms disappeared. . . . We specifically inquire as to the use of oral contraceptives in all young women we see with rheumatic complaints. . . ."

Two English doctors reported on a twenty-seven-year-old woman who had been on one pill for seven months and then switched to another brand. Two weeks later her upper arms and legs started to ache painfully. The pains disappeared two weeks after she stopped the Pill. She tried to go back on the Pill a few months later, but experienced the same pains again. After she discontinued the drug, the pain gradually subsided.

"I couldn't move my knee"

Ms. Geri B., a young attorney, stopped the Pill within two months of getting rheumatic pains. She started taking the Pill in September. Just before Christmas, she related, "I woke up one morning to find I couldn't move my knee, I couldn't get out of bed. The pain was unbearable, but it went away in about an hour.

"It happened fairly often, say three to five times a week. Once it took almost two hours to go away. Usually the pain was in the right knee, but sometimes in the left. Never in both at once. The stiffness in my knee got very bothersome and in February I stopped the Pill." Since then, Geri reported, she has had only two similar attacks, and both of these occurred shortly after she stopped the Pill.

The Royal College of Physicians in London reports that the Pill may sometimes have a protective effect against rheumatoid arthritis. The British doctors point out that pregnancy also relieves arthritis in some women, although why this should be is still unclear. What is clear is that the Pill has some effect on the immune responses in a woman's blood, which can affect her chances, one way or another, of developing arthritis. Such a basic bodily change is potentially quite dangerous in the long run.

Menstrual disturbances are such a common side effect that they are almost taken for granted. They include lighter periods, heavier periods, missed periods, and spotting or staining ("breakthrough bleeding"). A study by researchers in Czechoslovakia showed that 45 percent of the women observed there reported one or more of these changes.

Breakthrough bleeding is one of the most common reasons cited by women who give up the Pill. One suburban housewife told us, "It was so embarrassing. I never knew when a spot would show on my dress. When I reached the stage where I was afraid to drive over to the shopping center without putting in a tampon first, I decided to quit. My husband didn't like it either. Some men don't mind, I suppose. But he's sort of squeamish."

Certain vaginal infections are very common. Most Pill users get them only occasionally, but find them most unpleasant. One woman described it as having "horrible, white, peeling blobs."

Most clear up quickly with medication, but some are "intractable" as long as the patient remains on the Pill, and the treatment is usually rather unpleasant. Dermatologists are sometimes called upon to help treat difficult cases, and the *Archives of Dermatology* has reported that treatment may be only "temporarily effective" unless the Pill is discontinued.

The Pill was once considered an acceptable treatment for severe acne. A nineteen-year-old college student who works part-time in a drugstore and likes to think of himself as a man of the world told us, "I always keep my eye out for girls whose complexions clear up suddenly. I figure they may be on the Pill and I might luck into something." Many women do develop beautiful complexions; others, however, complain that theirs are ruined. A woman who developed bumpy skin after nine months on the Pill told us that the minute she walked into her dermatologist's office, he said, "You're on the Pill!"

Her bumpy skin cleared up after she stopped the Pill.

Other women find that the Pill's damage lingers on for months or even years. One concerned mother wrote us about her daughter, Lois, who has been fighting the Pill's aftereffects for longer than she took the Pill.

Lois apparently "suffered a staggering imbalance of testosterone, which has caused severe adult acne and an increase of body and facial hair. She has since run the gamut of dermatologists, endocrinologists, gynecologists, plastic surgeons, and electrolysis." Her mother reports that Lois was "treated with batteries of hormones, unguents, other treatments, and chauvinistic platitudes like 'I like hairy women.'" She is now taking a combination of hormones and antibiotics "on a long-term basis." Needless to say, both Lois and her mother are wondering what further effects those drugs will have.

One skin problem that usually cannot be reversed is discoloration. The affected areas may be as small and scattered as irregularly shaped moles or they may appear in the form of huge, ugly patches across the chin, cheeks, forehead, and nose. These nonreversible skin discolorations are among the most common side effects of the Pill. In a study performed at Scott Air Force Base in Illinois, 61 out of 212 Pill users (29 percent) suffered skin discolorations. Brunettes are more susceptible than blondes, and the incidence for them may be higher. A fatal skin cancer, malignant melanoma, has also been linked to the Pill (see Chapter 6).

Other side effects linked to beauty (and vanity) problems are weight changes and breast changes. Weight changes are not always in the wrong direction. One study of 1,160 Pill users revealed that half of them gained weight, a third lost weight, and the rest reported no change.

Most women are delighted when their breasts become larger, but at times an increase in size is no joy.

Rhoda K., a nurse who lives and works in Houston, started

taking the Pill a couple of weeks before her marriage. Her doctor said, "I'll give you the Pill, because I think it's great for newlyweds. No muss, no fuss, no bother. But in six months or so, when you and your husband have adjusted sexually, I want you to come back and let me give you something else. I don't think it's a good idea to stay on it too long."

Rhoda spent most of her European honeymoon resting with an ice pack on each breast. "For the entire month that I was on the Pill, I felt pain and soreness in my breasts," she reports. "They became so enlarged that most days I couldn't even fasten my bra to get dressed and go out sightseeing." She improved as soon as she came home and was fitted for a diaphragm.

Loss of hair and teeth

When a woman starts losing her hair, she is more likely to turn to her hairdresser for help than to her doctor. One New York coiffeur with a jet-set clientele told us, "I've seen at least thirty women who are losing their hair and I suspect they're all on the Pill. I *know* some of them are.

"When a girl comes in and tells me her hair is coming out, I immediately ask if she's on the Pill, especially if I know she hasn't had a lot of hair coloring or straightening. And when they say, 'Yes,' I tell them they should go see their doctor right away."

There is even a good chance that some long-term Pill users will end up losing some of their teeth. The Pill is often reported to create gum problems. Many dentists will not use it. One New York dentist, who specializes in gum surgery, told us that she always asks new women patients, "Are you on the Pill?" If her examination suggests that periodontal treatment is indicated, she also advises a switch to some other form of birth control.

The type of gum trouble experienced by Pill users—spongy gums, gingivitis (inflammation with bleeding), mobile teeth—is very similar to that suffered during pregnancy. But there is one big difference. Women who are on the Pill require much more time to heal. The gum specialist whom we interviewed estimated that two or three out of every ten patients who were on the Pill suffered from gum trouble, either caused or aggravated by the Pill. Often the delicate tissues around the necks of the teeth have become infected. When surgery is necessary, it takes normal patients a month to six weeks to heal. Pill users may take as long as six months. A significant number of patients who had been on the Pill and stopped began to heal more rapidly after oral contraceptives were discontinued. Others continued to have trouble for considerable time.

One case was described to this specialist by a periodontist from Lubbock, Texas, who had a Pill-using patient who needed eighteen months to heal after gum surgery. One of the New York doctor's own patients was a twenty-four-year-old schoolteacher who had entered treatment when her gums became inflamed, spongy, and painful and began bleeding excessively. The dentist immediately asked her if she was on the Pill. She said she had been taking it off and on for almost two years to regulate her periods. The improvement in her gums was dramatic when she stopped the Pill. The dentist originally thought she would have to perform surgery, but this proved unnecessary.

This doctor makes a point of telling patients with daughters what she has observed in the mouths of women who take the Pill. She suggests that the mothers advise their daughters to consider other means of birth control. And the *British Medical Journal* has carried an editorial cautioning, "We should add to our list of warnings given to the patient for whom oral contraceptives are prescribed that she will need regular dental care."

As Dr. Sumner Kalman, a Stanford University pharmacologist, has pointed out, the effect of a drug on the body is highly personal. How a woman feels about her reaction is highly personal, too. For example, we interviewed half a dozen women who had developed disfiguring little spider veins in their legs and thighs. Four stopped the Pill immediately. One of the four, a cocktail waitress in a club where the abbreviated costumes of the waitresses are one of the attractions, was extremely angry. She considered that the spider veins directly affected her earning power. The two women who stayed on the Pill despite the spider veining had different motivations.

Ramona F. couldn't care less. She lives and works in New York's Greenwich Village and enjoys the freedom of being single. She explained, "My legs were never my glory. They're too fat. I was nineteen when I started on the Pill, and these veins broke out immediately. My doctor told me to stop. He gave me an IUD, but it didn't work. I had to have two abortions in one year. After the second the doctor said, 'Well, if you're not going to use a diaphragm, I'd better put you back on the Pill. We'll try a different brand this time.' I've been back on the Pill for two years. I got a few more veins at the beginning, but then they quieted down."

Denise S. is a divorcée in her thirties and a copywriter in a large Chicago advertising agency. She hides her veins with a special cream. She is husband-hunting and is worried that continued use of the Pill will worsen the situation, but she feels it is the best contraceptive for her way of life. Every time she shaves her legs, she examines them carefully in a three-way mirror to be sure the veins are not getting worse.

Facial hair is another occasional side effect and one that most women find intolerable. Yet we interviewed one woman who likes the Pill so much that she stays with it, even though she has what she describes as a "real beard and mustache" and has to undergo extensive facial electrolysis every three months.

An Australian doctor has reported that the Pill can affect hearing. Dr. A. B. K. Watkins, writing in the *Medical Journal of Australia*, said that some of his patients on the Pill, just like some pregnant women, developed abnormalities of the Eustachian tubes, which lead from the back of the throat to the middle ear. As a result, the woman's own breathing can cause "a roaring in her ears."

The Pill has even been known to affect the voice levels of professional singers. In Copenhagen, where musical standards are high, the Royal Theater's own physician decides whether or not an artist will perform. In at least two cases the doctor kept sopranos in the wings. The Royal Society of Medicine was advised of "two cases of vocal changes in sopranos" that resulted in "loss of the two highest tones after only one week's use of oral contraceptives." The Danish doctor strongly advised women singers against the Pill because of the "virilizing changes" resulting in lower notes that occur following even moderate doses. This was of interest to impresarios the world over, because it had become fairly common practice for a singer to request the Pill to delay menstruation until after a major first-night performance. Another sour note sounded by the Pill.

CHAPTER 12

Depression and the Pill

Women psychiatrists were among the first doctors to stop using birth control pills. Finely tuned to emotional feedback, they did not take long to notice certain adverse reactions in themselves and their daughters, patients, and friends. The effects that were the most obvious ranged from suicidal and even murderous tendencies to increased irritability and tearfulness.

Some reactions, such as irritability, constant fatigue, and crying jags, are relatively minor in that they affect the quality of life, but not life itself. We will discuss these in the following chapter.

In London, the Royal College of Physicians found that the rate of suicide among Pill-takers was two to three times as high as among other women. They also noted that those who take the Pill are twice as likely to die from accidents. Death because of accident may be simply accidental, but in some cases it is a form of suicide. The woman becomes accident-prone as an unconscious means of self-destruction. Others may find that they are accident-prone because of a general anxiety or nervousness.

British researchers have established that *one out of every three* Pill users who were studied showed depressive personality changes. And three out of fifty who were studied intensively became suicidal. Some researchers have opined that suicide—not blood clots or cardiovascular disease—may actually be the leading cause of Pill-related deaths.

As with so many of the Pill's effects, it is hard to separate the physical and the psychological reasons for depression. Some women are afraid for their own health or resentful of their husbands or lovers. Still others may want a baby and resent the circumstances that lead them to use contraceptives. Still others may be suffering from the ambivalence of a woman who both does and does not want a child.

When the metabolic effects of the Pill are considered, however, it is no wonder that so many women become depressed while taking it. The Pill causes several vitamin deficiencies and a general imbalance in the woman's nutrients (see Chapter 14). "These would be expected to involve a general malaise and depression," according to Australian researchers Michael and Maxine Briggs. In particular, the Pill's effects on vitamins B_1, B_6, and B_{12} would be expected to have psychiatric effects.

In pioneering research performed by Dr. Victor Wynn and his associates in London, thirty-nine women who had developed depression while on the Pill were closely evaluated. Nineteen had severe B_6 deficiency and improved significantly when treated with 40 mg daily of the vitamin. (B_6, or pyridoxine, has an essential though imperfectly understood effect on mood and the chemistry of the brain.) All told, about half of depressed Pill users reveal marked B_6 deficiency, and all of these respond quite dramatically to the supplement. Most long-term Pill users develop *some* B_6 deficiency, but if it is only moderate, supplements do not counter the emotional distress.

Dr. Wynn is no loose advocate of vitamin supplementation, for, as he points out, at high dosages vitamins start to have pharmacological effects. To avoid imbalances, it is desirable to take the entire vitamin B complex and vitamin C as well along with the B_6.

The best treatment for Pill-caused depression is to stop the Pill, but when this is not possible, pyridoxine is probably a safer alternative than antidepressants.

Another physical effect of the Pill that might induce depression involves an enzyme known as MAO. Oral contraceptives produce a high level of MAO activity in the womb. For this reason, some of the drugs given to depressed patients inhibit MAO activity.

A variety of emotional symptoms have been observed in Pill users. Some women become agitated and disorganized. Some can't sleep. Some withdraw and become indifferent to their families and surroundings. Some Pill users suffer from several of these symptoms. Or they may crash their automobiles or set "accidental" fires. These are just some of the ways for a person to signal that she is incapable of taking care of herself or anyone else. When women with such symptoms seek help from physicians and psychiatrists, they often describe themselves as "hysterical" or "on the verge of a nervous breakdown."

An even greater number suffer from being deeply and specifically depressed—not in any casual sense of the term, but darkly and sometimes suicidally. They feel sad, hopeless, helpless, guilty, unworthy, ashamed, enervated, constipated. Some lose their appetite; others eat compulsively. Their nights are long and wakeful, and they greet the first light of dawn with a feeling of overwhelming hopelessness that makes them think: "Oh, my God, how can I get through another day?"

During the day, they can't concentrate. They report that they may read through a recipe or magazine article and then realize that they have not the faintest idea of what they read.

Decisions often become impossible, even if it is only a question such as: "Should I buy apples or pears?"

Occasionally these depression victims are also possessed by feelings of anxiety or even terror. One woman told us, "I was going to the movies and I was suddenly gripped by a fear that the buildings would topple over on me. The world seemed rotten through and through and about to come to an end. I grabbed my husband's arm. I could hardly put one foot in front of the other. It was early evening and the sun was setting. It looked ominous and terrifying. I believe I could have collected myself if the movie had been a comedy or a spy story. But it was a 1940s Bette Davis movie—a real five-handkerchief special. I started to weep. First just a little, like some of the other women in the theater. Then I was sobbing great horrible sobs. People turned around and looked at me. My husband led me out, hailed a taxi, and took me home. Then he called the doctor."

"She talked about 'ending it all'"

Relief comes—if it comes—in the evening. And only briefly. There is the realization: "I made it. I got through another day." These are typical symptoms of depression.

Psychiatrists noticed the Pill-caused increase in the incidence of depression not only because they observed changes among their families and friends but also because they usually see patients with considerable regularity and are familiar with the details of their lives, emotions, and personalities. Sometimes the depression was mild. In other cases the personality changes were swift and severe.

A Manhattan psychiatrist told us, "My fights with the gynecologists began in 1963. I'd been seeing one patient twice a week for two years. I knew her better than her mother did. Perhaps better than I know my own wife. She was tough as nails. A remarkable woman. The oldest of eight children. Her father had been an alcoholic. She'd fought her way to the top as a fashion model. She was seeing me because of her problems with men. The only men who attracted her were weak men like her father. She was aware of this and didn't want to lead a life like her mother. She's one of the most sensible patients I ever had. Exploitive? Yes. Neurotic? A little. Depressed? Never.

"Eight days after this patient went on the Pill, she arrived for her appointment and wept through the whole session. The same thing happened the next time. And the next. Her speech was slowing. Her usually perky walk had become a kind of shuffle. She talked about 'giving up' and 'ending it all.'

"I suggested that she get off the Pill. We'd see what happened then. She did. The next time I saw her she was her old self. But then came the first in a series of calls from her gynecologist. In essence what he had to say was 'You stick to your own unraveling or whatever it is you do, and let me take care of *my* knitting. Birth control is not a psychiatrist's province.' That doctor has changed his tune, though. Now he sends me patients for treatment for Pill-caused depressions."

Another psychiatrist, this time practicing in the Midwest, told of Bertha D., who was referred to him by her family doctor because of depression and irritability. Her personality had changed so radically that the family doctor was even more alarmed about her children than he was about her. Mrs. D., who had always been affectionate with her children, a gentle disciplinarian, had given her five-year-old daughter a black eye for not standing still while her hair was being braided.

"I made a diagnosis of depression," the psychiatrist told us, "and prescribed suitable medication. She kept on with the Pill. She didn't improve . . . except for the five days in every cycle when she was off the Pill. When she resumed, her psychiatric symptoms reappeared. After several months of this, she stopped the Pill. Within a few weeks her fury, her emotional withdrawal, and her crying spells were nearly gone. A month later she felt like her own self."

A gynecologist who spotted the emotional side effects of the Pill early, Dr. John R. McCain, testified at the U. S. Senate's 1970 Nelson hearings on the Pill. He told the senators that emotional or psychiatric problems are among the most potentially dangerous complications.

Most of the patients in whom Dr. McCain observed adverse psychiatric reactions were women with a medical problem who were taking the Pill to cure it. Three became suicidal: two of them within the first two weeks of Pill use, the third in her fourth month.

One thirty-two-year-old patient telephoned Dr. McCain. She told him that for over a week she had been dreaming of killing herself and that she was terribly afraid she would commit suicide. She had been on the Pill for fourteen days in an attempt to control a menstrual irregularity. The doctor advised her to stop taking the Pill, and she soon returned to her normal personality. In three years Dr. McCain treated seven other patients with severe psychiatric symptoms that were triggered by the Pill.

Discontinuing the Pill is enough for some patients, but others require vitamin B_6 therapy or psychiatric treatment—not only antidepressant drugs, but sometimes even shock treatment and hospitalization.

Dr. Frank J. Ayd, Jr., author of *Recognizing the Depressed Patient*, says, "I have seen enough cases of severe depression from the Pill so that, on this basis alone, I would never give the Pill to my wife or daughters." Almost all the psychiatrists we interviewed felt the same way.

In the *American Journal of Obstetrics and Gynecology*, Dr. Francis J. Kane reported that more than 50 percent of 139 relatively young, well-educated women perceived changes in themselves, most often of an adverse nature, after starting the Pill. Depression occurred in 34 percent of this group, which was studied at the University of North Carolina at Chapel Hill.

At the University of Lund in Sweden, Drs. A. Nilsson and P. S. Almgren studied 165 pregnant women. In addition to taking a careful pre-pregnancy psychiatric history of all these patients, the investigators also observed and tested them throughout pregnancy. After delivery 54 women selected the Pill, while 104 others selected different contraceptives.

The results were startling. A significantly higher frequency of psychiatric symptoms showed up in women using oral contraceptives, even though there was no difference between the two groups in respect to past psychiatric symptoms, during pregnancy or before. The Pill users and non–Pill users were also similar in social background and other possibly significant factors. Reporting this research in the *British Medical Journal*, the doctors concluded that the psychiatric side effects of the Pill can presumably be ascribed to hormonal factors.

A report by a team of British investigators also appeared in the *British Medical Journal*. Drs. Ellen Grant and John Pryse-Davies studied a total of 797 women who received one or more of 34 different oral contraceptives. Many of the women reported mood disturbances and simultaneous vascular side effects. Of 136 women taking a certain brand, two became so depressed that they actually did attempt suicide.

When pills fight other pills

Before the magnitude of the Pill's effects on the body was generally recognized, quite a few doctors speculated that the blame for Pill-induced emotional crises might lie more in the user than in the chemicals. It was pointed out that some women had "magical expectations" of the Pill. Some hoped that it would cure frigidity and were bitterly disappointed when it failed. A psychoanalyst, Dr. Natalie Shainess, points out that the Pill has brought many couples to realize that they did not care for each other sexually; it was not just an old-fashioned pre-Pill contraceptive or fear of pregnancy that kept them apart, as each had pretended.

Other wives bitterly resented their husbands for forcing them to assume responsibility for contraception, especially with a contraceptive that had so many side effects. Repression of such a rage could lead to depression. It is now generally believed that while many Pill-associated depressions are caused by hormones alone, others are triggered by a combination of hormones and psychological factors or, in still other cases, by psychological factors alone.

The Food and Drug Administration has included suicide among the causes of Pill deaths received by the agency. In the labeling information that Pill manufacturers must supply to doctors, one precaution reads: "Patients with a history of psychic depression should be carefully observed and the drug discontinued if the depression recurs to a serious degree."

Conscientious doctors not only question a patient about depressive tendencies but also about any family history of depression before putting her on the Pill, because hereditary factors can be significant.

It is also a great tragedy, Dr. Ayd told us, that some physicians still give patients tranquilizers to counteract Pill-caused psychiatric symptoms. Some drugs, taken in combination, produce untoward effects in some people. The combination of the Pill and certain psychiatric drugs can produce a broad range of dangerous and unpleasant effects. Among these are tremor and rigidity, as in Parkinson's disease; an inability to sit still; acute twisting of the body so that it is bent like a bow; tremendous weight gain, far beyond what the Pill alone had produced; and increased interference with sugar metabolism.

"It needs to be emphasized," Dr. Ayd concluded, "that if you give a patient one drug and counteract it with another, there is a rising curve of adverse reactions."

Again and again we heard of cases where the inability of busy practitioners to keep up with the volume and variety of negative scientific reports about the Pill was potentially threatening to human life. One gynecologist told us of his grave concern for his daughter, a young married woman with one child, and normally a happy person. The Pill triggered off a severe depression in her and she went to a psychiatrist. He took her off the Pill and she got better immediately. After the birth of her son her own gynecologist allowed her to resume a different brand of the Pill. At last report she appeared to be doing well. But her father, who is a medical school professor, felt he knew more about pharmacology than her doctor. The father told us:

"He's a competent and busy man, a fine practitioner—but he lacks the time to read that I have. We teachers have to keep up, you know, much more than the average practitioner. My daughter's doctor may well be more skilled at delivering babies than I am—in fact I'm sure he is—but I know more about the pharmacological effects of the Pill. I'm afraid that once a woman's body has shown such a marked adverse response to the hormones—it was really a bad depression, you know, she tried to take her life—this is a warning that she may respond that way again. Basically, the chemicals in all the pills are a good deal alike and I'm just afraid that this time the depression will take longer to develop. Her mother and I are quite anxious. We've pleaded with her and spoken with her gynecologist, but what else can we do?"

"I wasn't the person they knew"

A Houston psychiatrist told us of patients with whom "the Pill pulls the plug on severe depression which may have been smoldering for some time."

In Los Angeles, Doris H., a twenty-eight-year-old secretary and doctor's daughter, began taking the Pill. "By summer," she related, "my friends were telling me I wasn't the happy person they knew. I was depressed all the time.

"The doctor who treated me for a case of dysentery insisted I stop taking the Pill. He thought it was from the birth control pills. I chose to believe that it was a bug from traveling overseas. I did stop taking them and, miraculously, the depression slowly left. I started to be *me* again."

But Doris had still not learned her lesson. Two years later she again started taking birth control pills. The depression began creeping back. This time, she said, "It was an immobilizing depression. I couldn't pull myself out of it. No influence in the world could bring me to a normal level. I was crying at least once a day. I would say to myself, 'This is stupid; what am I crying about?'"

The depression continued in varying degrees for the next two years. Then Doris discovered a tumor in her breast. It was benign.

She continued: "The doctor who took the tumor out decided it was the result of the Pill. He had seen the same structure in other women who had taken the Pill, which left him with no doubt at all. He forbade me, under penalty of another tumor, from taking birth control pills.

"There was an almost immediate end to the depression this time. Within two to four weeks it was gone. This time I was convinced that the Pill had been the direct cause. If I had to, I might risk another benign tumor, but the depression was more than I could ever stand again."

CHAPTER 13

Irritability and the Pill

The nutritional deficiencies (see Chapter 14) and metabolic effects of the Pill may cause irritability and nervousness as well as depression. Some women become so irritable that their husbands, friends, and children find it impossible to get along with them.

"When I was on the Pill, I hardly ever got up off the couch except to slap one of the children." So said a psychiatrist's wife when she phoned us from Chicago. She had heard we were writing a book about the Pill, and she wanted us to know her story and why her doctor husband had asked her to stop taking the Pill.

"As I look back on it," she said, "I was always irritable and tired. Like I'd been on my pregnancies, only worse. I would lie there on that couch and take one catnap after another. Getting supper at night was a real effort.

"I never felt like going out. I was going to stick it out in the hope that I would eventually feel better, but my husband said that it looked to him like I was never going to get beyond the first trimester. That's what it was really like. Like perpetual early pregnancy. So I stopped."

A man doesn't have to be a psychiatrist to make the diagnosis when his wife is less lovable on the Pill. In Canada, the Toronto *Globe and Mail* reported that one young husband took his wife to the doctor to find out what could be causing the drastic change in her disposition. The doctor traced the change back to the time the woman began taking the Pill. When the couple got home, the husband took his wife's birth control pills and threw them out into the snow.

Dr. Philip Ball, a Mayo-trained internist-diagnostician in Muncie, Indiana, was among the first to warn about mood changes on the Pill. He documented eleven of his own cases, where fatigue, irritability, depression, and a lack of libido were cured by discontinuing the Pill.

One of Dr. Ball's patients had been taking the Pill for two years when she consulted him for a long-standing fatigue. "She had also gained considerable weight and felt herself to be twenty-five pounds above desirable weight. . . . She wanted to lose weight, then discontinue the contraceptive, and have another baby—in that order. She felt that she couldn't lose [weight] so long as she took the contraceptive pill and couldn't afford to get pregnant as overweight as she was. . . . Here was a female who was fat, fatigued, pigmented, infertile, and confused as to what to do next. I told her to stop all pills."

More than 150 cases

Dr. Ball commented that he did not believe that contraceptive pills were responsible for "all of the fat, fatigued, fussy, fluid-filled females in the country." He concluded: "Maybe they are only causing one fourth of the problems, but this is too much."

A year after his article had appeared, we interviewed Dr. Ball who told us that he had seen more than 150 women with similar complaints since he had decided to write it. "The worst offense in my book is to give the Pill to a bride. She gets married and goes to live in a different city. She doesn't like the city. She doesn't like married life, doesn't like the apartment, and doesn't like *him*. I've seen women who thought it was the wrong city and the wrong husband, but when they stopped the Pill everything was rosy."

One young woman who thought everything was going wrong for her when she was on the Pill told us, "I turned into a fishwife." This was Elsie E., an English teacher with a two-year-old son. Her husband, Jeff, was working for his doctor's degree in psychology. Elsie started taking the Pill three months after her baby was born. When her doctor learned about our book, he suggested that we talk to Elsie about her experience with the Pill.

"My husband ran out of patience with me," she said. "I just couldn't seem to handle anything."

As she unfolded the story of her experience, it was evident that Elsie made enormous demands upon herself. She tried to be a good teacher, a good wife and mother, a good cook, and a good housekeeper simultaneously. And she was all those things until she started on the Pill. It not only made her teaching life miserable; it came close to breaking up her marriage.

"I thought the principal of my school was out to fire me," she recalled. "I thought he lurked behind every door waiting for me to foul things up. But he didn't. He didn't feel that way about me at all. He knew from the way the children reacted to me that I was succeeding. I was the one who couldn't believe it.

"I was sure the other teachers hated me, too. I was a modern teacher. I wanted to teach grammar through structure and sentence patterns and so forth. I was not forceful or dynamic enough to get the older teachers to agree to this. I took it all personally. I couldn't see that this was only an academic disagreement. I thought they didn't like *me*.

"And I sought the adoration of the children. They all had to like me, although I know that that's absolutely impossible. I was really hurt if I ever heard one of my students say anything bad about me. I took it personally.

"But when I was on the Pill, I felt persecuted all the time. It was terrible for my husband, because here he was, trying to finish up his degree, and I never gave him a moment's peace at home. Like, if I were cooking and I dropped a spoon, I could sit down and cry about it for an hour. I was plagued by the house, too. If anything was out of place, it was terrible.

"Jeff and I used to sit and talk about it. He'd say, 'You're sure not the woman I married.' And there were times when, intellectually, I could admit it. But I was powerless to do anything about it. I was just in an emotional corner. I didn't know how to get out.

"We were fortunate, because when we got married we were in Germany without family, without friends. I learned to speak German so I could talk to my neighbors. My husband and I were very, very close. This is probably the only thing that kept us together when I was on the Pill. We knew what we had had together.

"We blamed the fact that I had turned into such a bitch on the fact that I had not adjusted to motherhood. For a year, it was just the two of us alone—and then we had this bawling kid around. But the way it worked, I turned all my love to the baby, and that was the last thing I really wanted to do. I always felt that parenthood is something you work to get fired from in twenty years. But I just wrapped my whole life around our little boy, Mike. When he was going through the normal crisis of being upset when I was away, I made it worse. I decided that I should never leave him. I wouldn't even have a baby-sitter come for an evening. We never went out. It got to the point that he wouldn't play outside unless I was with him.

"He's getting out of that now, thank goodness. Lots of times he says things like, 'You'll always take care of me, won't you?' And I say, 'No, Mike, I'll take care of you as long as you need me, but every day I want you to learn to take a little care of yourself. Mommy's job is only to take care of those things you can't do for yourself.' He's slowly getting over the notion that I am like a kangaroo whose pouch he can jump into if something goes wrong.

"And all this was the Pill. I'm not like that anymore," Elsie said, "and I wasn't like it before. I know myself pretty well. I like reinforcement. If I bake a fine pie, I like my husband to say 'That's a good pie.' But he doesn't have to go into a twenty-five-minute dissertation on how good it is. When I was on the Pill, if I didn't have constant praise, I thought it meant people hated me.

"Now I can take things in stride. It took about two months, though, after I stopped taking the Pill before I came back to acting normal."

"What's happening to me?"

Another young woman had a similar experience. In her case the general irritability was accompanied by physical symptoms that were serious enough to send her to her doctor, who promptly took her off the Pill. This was Bettina L. She was twenty-three when we interviewed her. She was born in the Netherlands and came to this country when she was thirteen. She was married at twenty-one when still in college. She told us, "I started on the Pill right after I got married. I got a little bit sick to my stomach when I first started, but . . . I really didn't think about it much.

"Well, along in the summertime, I started having terrible cramps in my legs. Especially at night. My husband would have to get up at night with me, because my legs were cramped. I never had this before. Never.

"And then it started. I couldn't eat without vomiting right after. And the headaches. And I was so tired. I could just lie down in the afternoon and sleep. My legs were swollen.

"Thank goodness, my husband is very understanding. While I was on the Pill, I felt like another person, because I was always depressed. I thought, 'My goodness, what's happening to me?'

"So I went to the doctor. He asked me to stop taking the Pill. And I did, that very day. After a week, everything disappeared. All the symptoms went away. I felt like myself again. And, like I said, thank God, my husband is understanding. I imagine if some girls got married and felt ill and cranky all the time I did, I think it could break a marriage very easily."

Young women are not the only ones who suffer personality

changes. Kay D., a television actress in her thirties, gave up the Pill because "I was making scenes in the grocery stores. There were plenty of stores in my neighborhood where I'd thrown such a tantrum that I was ashamed to go back. I finally figured out that I was in trouble if I could get so mad just because the girl in the supermarket wasn't punching the cash register fast enough."

In some women the personality changes caused by the Pill are almost immediately apparent. In others the changes emerge slowly and almost imperceptibly. Didi S. stopped taking the Pill because it had caused recurrent fungus infections that the doctor could not cure. Shortly afterward she realized that she was a "different woman." She told us, "All of a sudden, my kids' manners were better. The flowers in my backyard looked prettier. And I realized that my sister-in-law means well. She really does."

Didi told us that she hadn't realized that she had been affected psychically by the Pill until after she stopped taking it. "I used to boast that it hadn't affected me at all," she said. "I was just slightly more uptight than usual. Like the day before my period. I always seemed to feel that way. I guess you can say, it made me perpetually premenstrual."

"I'm much more relaxed"

Like Didi, Karen P. didn't notice any change in her personality until she stopped the Pill. "I didn't stop for any special reason. It was just that my husband and I kept reading about it and we became convinced that the risks outweighed the benefits. We managed before with the condom—and we're doing it again. But about six months after I stopped, my husband was in the kitchen for a snack and he called out to me in great surprise, 'Hey, you've still got all those glasses we bought last summer!' He was right. I hadn't been breaking any glasses lately. The reason he was so surprised is that while I was on the Pill I went through almost a whole set of dishes, and I couldn't begin to count the glasses I broke. The Pill, I realized, had made me feel tense, and when I was tense I was clumsy. I know I'm much more relaxed now."

Such cases are by no means unusual. Dr. William A. Cantrell, professor of psychiatry at Baylor University College of Medicine, told us that the most common problem he saw among his Pill-using patients was the "mimicking of premenstrual tension, which is more or less continuous. They become anxious, depressed, jittery."

In London, a Harley Street specialist told us of a young woman, engaged to be married, who became so moody, irritable, tense, and tired on the Pill that she decided she didn't really want to marry her young man. They broke up and she returned to a life of celibacy without the Pill. It wasn't long before it dawned on her that the trouble had been the Pill, not the young man. She is now happily married to him, but is not on the Pill.

In Sweden, we learned of the case of Elisabeth A., a nurse in a small town who began taking the Pill when she was thirty-six. After two months she began to suffer from severe headaches and became so tired that she applied for sick leave and stayed home. Her head throbbed so badly that she stayed in a darkened room much of the time and was unable to read or do housecleaning chores. Finally, without consulting her doctor, she stopped taking the Pill, and the headaches and fatigue disappeared. Her husband was a pilot; the couple had a seven-year-old daughter, a pleasant home, and a happy circle of friends. Peace was restored.

Then, two years later, Mrs. A. decided to start up on the Pill again. Two and a half months later she began to grow irritable, to fight with her husband, strike her daughter, and cry constantly with no provocation. After a few days she became deeply depressed, stayed home, and didn't want to see or talk to anybody. Her doctor told her the Pill might be to blame. He advised her to stop taking it. She did. She gradually began to feel better, went back to work some weeks later, and has sworn off the Pill for good.

"A *very dangerous medicament*"

In addition to the hormone-linked irritability, tears, fatigue, and so on, there are other tensions based on what psychiatrists term reality factors. One reality factor, according to Dr. Francis J. Kane, the University of North Carolina psychiatrist, is "body damage." Some women fear that the Pill may be harming their body. Typically, a woman may think she is not affected by the frightening stories she may read or hear about the Pill; yet if she is on the Pill, she worries. Infantile omnipotence ("It can't happen to me") may not be quite strong enough to prevent this subconscious worrying—unless a woman is indeed infantile.

Many doctors who are in favor of the Pill argue that its emotional side effects are caused by such reality factors as the fears of women, not by the Pill's hormones. The dilemma, of course, is that the Pill's hormonal effects are themselves a crucial reality of the Pill—perhaps the most crucial reality of all.

The problem of reality, and the human response to it, was highlighted when a twenty-nine-year-old British housewife died of pulmonary embolism and bleeding in the brain. Professor J. M. Webster, the Home Office pathologist who looked into this case, concluded: "I have no hesitation whatsoever in saying that this young woman died from the effects of taking what is in my opinion a very dangerous medicament, which is called the Pill." The Deputy Coroner, P. J. Monkman, was also emphatic when recording his verdict. He said, "It is quite clear that the Pill was the cause of death."

British newspapers reported the case prominently, especially because of the comments by Professor Webster and Mr. Monkman. This prompted Dr. Stanley Way, a gynecologist at Queen Elizabeth Hospital in Gateshead, to charge that the newspapers had probably "scared [many women] out of their wits." Dr. Way may have been right. But did not the news media have an obligation to cover the case and didn't British women have the right to know that experts thought the Pill was "a very dangerous medicament"?

Dr. Way was probably overestimating the power of the press and underestimating the practicality of the female. A study by the Demographic Research and Training Center in Chembur, India, established that three out of four women on the Pill in Bombay stopped taking it by the end of two years, not because they were scared by newspaper reports but because of side effects. Other studies indicate that one woman in three gives up the Pill by the end of the first year and one woman in two gives it up by the end of the second year—for reasons other than the desire to become pregnant. Many authorities believe that the dropout rate may actually be higher and that psychological distress is one of the main reasons for discontinuing. This means that thousands of women have decided there is no percentage in feeling pregnant or premenstrual forever. Or as Dr. Philip Ball asked one young patient, "Why go through life feeling miserable when, with a little more care and a little more trouble, you can be very healthy and have a joyful life?"

CHAPTER 14

The Pill and Nutrition

One of the least-known facts about the Pill is that it makes a mockery of a good diet. Today many doctors are aware that the Pill affects just about every cell in the body and interferes with basic bodily functions. But most are unaware that the Pill creates deficiencies of vitamins C, thiamine (B_1), riboflavin (B_2), pyridoxine (B_6), B_{12}, folic acid, and E, as well. The Pill also depletes essential trace minerals, including zinc and magnesium. It mysteriously increases a woman's plasma vitamin A, copper, and niacin; it is possible, too, that Pill users need less iron.

In fact, there are only four major nutrients that may be unaltered by the Pill: vitamin D, K, pantothenic acid, and biotin.

These nutritional alterations are suspected of playing a role in some of the Pill's side effects, including changes in the cervix, depression, irritability, birth defects, susceptibility to infections, and post-Pill menstrual disorders.

Certain of the Pill's side effects might be dependent to some extent upon diet. Women in developing countries who have very-low-fat diets, for example, would not be expected to develop cardiovascular disease at the same rate as women in Western nations whose diets are relatively high in meats and other fats. The same might be true of the Pill's effects on glucose tolerance: those who consume a great deal of sugar might run a very high risk of developing prediabetic states while on the Pill.

Women who must take the Pill for medical reasons, women who are determined to take it as a contraceptive, and women who are suffering from its aftermath can take some simple steps to compensate for its nutritional ravages. Vitamin therapy often alleviates some Pill problems, particularly depression and the infertility associated with the Pill. Vitamin therapy is also useful in reversing the Pill's adverse effects on the cervix, and in some cases may prevent surgery.

The vitamin regimen, however, must be carefully thought out, since the Pill causes excesses as well as deficiencies. An excess of vitamin A, for example, may cause birth defects and emotional disturbances. If a woman stops the Pill to have a baby and does not get her periods back, she should, perhaps, be careful to avoid taking vitamin A, which is included in most multivitamin supplements. At the same time, therapeutic doses of certain other vitamins, particularly folic acid, vitamin E, and vitamin B_6, might help her achieve normal fertility without the need for dangerous drugs.

Vitamin B_6 (pyridoxine)

B_6 is undervalued by most professionals, but it is one of the most essential vitamins. It affects the state of mind, nerves, hormonal balance, sexuality, and reproduction, as well as the skin. The recommended allowance of 2 mg (milligrams) is too low for many women, since people differ in how their bodies use this nutrient. Those who suffer from metabolic disorders such as diabetes, hypoglycemia, celiac disease, and some cases of water retention and overweight may need more B_6. The same is true of anyone who is nervous, depressed, or suffering from severe premenstrual symptoms, skin problems, or tooth decay. After C, B_6 might be the vitamin that does the most to make other vitamins "work."

This vitamin's association with depression was proved by researchers working with women who took the Pill. Victor Wynn, a British endocrinologist, leads a team studying various metabolic disorders. As reported in Chapter 12, he and his colleagues discovered that 40 mg daily of vitamin B_6 often cures Pill-related depression.

Even more B_6—as much as 50 to 100 mg a day—is indicated for women who test out as "chemical diabetics" while taking the Pill. Women who find themselves infertile after stopping the Pill might wish briefly to try doses as high as 100 to 800 mg daily. In 1979 Drs. Joel Hargrove and Guy Abraham told the American Fertility Society that such megadoses cured 12 out of 14 infertile patients.*

B_6 tends to be expensive when it is extracted and synthesized. Roger Williams, who in 1933 discovered and named pantothenic acid, claims that most vitamin supplements do not contain much B_6 because of its cost. Women who choose multivitamins should look for brands that contain at least 5 mg; for those with the symptoms of diabetes or hypoglycemia, who are depressed, or who fail to conceive or menstruate, separate tablets of 50 mg or more may be advised.

The body's response to this or any other diet or vitamin regimen is an individual matter. The proper dose of any vitamin must ultimately be determined by the individual taking it. With B_6, nausea, severe premenstrual tension, and a lack of appetite in the morning may indicate a deficiency, as might the inability to remember dreams. Too much B_6, or too much at night, may cause insomnia, restlessness, or vivid dreams. It is possible that a person may need more B_6 while under stress, and less when the stress is relieved.

Folic acid

The effects of deficiencies of folic acid resemble those "female problems" common to Pill users, and some of them can be reversed by therapeutic doses of this vitamin.

A New York hematologist, John Lindenbaum, treated a number of Pill users who had abnormal Pap smears, indicating dangerous changes in the cervix. The three-week treatment in-

* Before self-prescribing doses of more than 100 mg, however, it would seem advisable to consult a nutritionist or knowledgeable physician.

volved enormous doses of folic acid—twenty-five times the RDA, or 10 mg daily. All of the Pap smears returned to normal, or near-normal, even while the women were still taking the Pill. Four of the women, however, discontinued their folic acid supplements and took the Pill for another three and one half years. In all four cases, Pap smears were again abnormal.

Pap smears are often abnormal in Pill users, and many doctors now take a wait-and-see attitude toward the cervical problems these women suffer. But other doctors are not that calm about these changes, which often resemble cancerous or precancerous conditions. Folate therapy might avert surgery for some women. It seems likely that it might also help women with other reproductive conditions caused by the Pill, including post-Pill infertility.

There is a close association between folic acid and estrogen. Without folic acid, the reproductive organs do not respond to estrogen. The cells and glands of all the reproductive organs are altered, and pregnancy is abnormal. Some of the most heartbreaking side effects of the Pill may be caused by its tendency to deplete folic acid.

A deficiency of this vitamin also causes other diseases, including a form of anemia that is sometimes fatal, and impairs the metabolism of other B vitamins, C, and nucleic acids. Those who are short of folic acid feel pain more sharply, suffer intestinal disturbances, and have decreased resistance to many infections.

It seems reasonable to suggest supplements to bring folic acid consumption to 400 mcg (the RDA) and possibly 800 mcg (0.8 mg) daily for women taking the Pill or recovering from it. Higher doses might be needed by those with cervicitis (inflammation of the cervix) or the glandular changes that result in abnormal Pap smears. Heavy drinkers have a greater need for folic acid than others, to correct deficiencies. Intake of more than 1 mg of folic acid daily may mask a B_{12} deficiency, which is most likely to occur in vegetarians or those who are unable to absorb B_{12}. For this reason, the FDA limited the amount of folic acid that may be contained in one pill to 0.8 mg. A folate-rich diet, perhaps with a supplement, is advisable for current or recent Pill users. Separate 0.4 or 0.8 mg folic acid supplements may be purchased at health food stores. (Most multivitamins do not contain this much folic acid.)

Foods rich in folates include liver—either beef, lamb, pork, or chicken, or desiccated liver; asparagus; spinach; wheat bran; dry beans; and yeast. Beef kidney has a moderate amount, and most other foods have small amounts. Nutritionists generally feel that it is very difficult to overdose on folic acid, since most of this vitamin is excreted within a day. Epileptics should avoid more than 1 mg a day, to forestall the possibility of an increased number of seizures. Occasionally an excess of folic acid may cause an allergic rash.

Vitamin C

The National Academy of Sciences established a Recommended Dietary Allowance of 50 to 60 milligrams of vitamin C daily for teenagers and adults, depending upon age. Many nutritionists, however, dispute the NAS, claiming that these allowances are far too low. Some have proposed dosages of several grams a day, even though such large doses might pose potential dangers.

One thing is clear: the Pill interferes with vitamin C utilization, and Pill users need more than other people. Smoking, air pollution, infection, illness, stress, late pregnancy, and aspirin-taking increase the need for C. A daily intake of 500 to 750 mg seems advisable for those who take the Pill, especially those who bruise easily or have spider veins or bleeding gums. Other signs of a vitamin C deficit in the body include intolerance to cold; aching joints; impaired maintenance of teeth, bones, and cartilage; weakness; listlessness; and rough skin.

As with some other vitamins, C affects other nutrients and helps other vitamins work better. It "conserves" most of the B vitamins, E, and A (and Pill users probably don't need to conserve A!). It also tends to deplete the body's B_{12} and folic acid (see below).

The body quickly rids itself of vitamin C, for reasons that are not well understood. Whatever C is appropriate for an individual woman should be divided into two or more doses and taken throughout the day. A woman who finds that 500 mg alleviates her symptoms should take 250 mg morning and night. Time-release capsules of C are now available, although they are costly.

At the Polytechnic of North London, nutritionists found that Pill-using patients who were given 3300 mg—an enormous dose—of vitamin C at night were still deficient by the following evening. The same group of researchers, however, also found that a group of Pill-takers avoided a deficiency of C by eating extra C-rich fresh fruits and vegetables for over a year.

Scientists at Mount Sinai Hospital in New York City recently reported that the vitamin C in oranges was much more biologically available in fresh orange juice than in either frozen or pasteurized orange juices. This is contrary to what nutritionists have believed, and taught, for many years.

There are some conditions—and some people—that respond better to vitamin C when it is accompanied by a controversial substance sometimes called vitamin P, or C complex. P is reportedly useful for gum problems, skin hemorrhages, and probably hot flashes. The need for vitamin P in humans has not been established, and many nutritionists would hesitate to call it a "vitamin." Yet vitamin P (the citrus bioflavonoids, rutin, and hesperidin) is found in nature, in the white part of the skin and the segments of citrus fruits and the white part of a green pepper. Vitamin C "complex" supplements are available and include both C and P.

For those who are already taking sufficient C, separate bioflavonoid supplements are sold. They should be used in proportion to the vitamin C intake: for each 500 mg of C, the usual therapeutic dose range is 100 to 200 mg of bioflavonoids, 50 mg of rutin, and 25 mg of hesperidin. The role of vitamin P has not been proved, but it may help prevent the destruction of C in the body.

Megadoses of vitamin C

Despite the body's ability to excrete vitamin C, those who take large doses run some risks, including those of diarrhea, kidney stones, and abdominal pain. One way to find out if a person is taking too much is to test her urine with a special dipstick, available at drugstores.

Vitamin C in large doses also creates a dependency, as does B_6. If the vitamin is stopped, blood levels of these vitamins fall below normal. In the case of C, this depletion may leave the person susceptible to colds and infections.

The interaction of aspirin and vitamin C is complicated. Since aspirin inhibits the transfer of C into the white blood cells, it would appear that extra C is needed when the patient is taking aspirin. However, the combination of aspirin and C affects the kidneys and may be dangerous. These effects have been noted with dosages of 3 to 5 grams of aspirin a day, along with high intakes of C. C also has complicated, and not always desirable, effects on the B vitamins, notably folic acid, and on the cervix. Since many Pill users develop problems in the cervix, they may have to walk a thin line to balance their C with folic acid.

Too much vitamin C washes out folic acid and destroys vitamin B_{12}. These two nutrients, so essential to mental and reproductive health, are also depleted by the Pill. Although C and B vitamins are combined in stress-formula vitamin pills, it may be advisable to take separate C and B tablets, at least three hours apart.

The threat of kidney stones can be diminished by cutting down on calcium, or by balancing calcium and magnesium intake. Since calcium is vital, and may be short in the diet, the calcium-magnesium combination equivalent to that in dolomite may be helpful.

Zinc

One of the best arguments the proponents of natural and organic foods have is the borderline deficiency of zinc in American diets. In current and former Pill users, this deficiency may
manifest itself as stretch marks, poor hair growth, fragile nails,
acne, joint pain, bruising, or the failure to menstruate.

Zinc deficiency exists because we grow our food in depleted
soil, overprocess it, and cook it poorly. In 1968 Dr. Frederick
Stare of the nutrition department of Harvard made a statement that the FDA, USDA, and other government agencies
are still quoting: "Fertilizers, regardless of type, do not
influence the nutrient composition of the plant in regard to its
content of protein, carbohydrates, or the various vitamins. . . ."
What Dr. Stare, who is known to some as the "Cornflakes Professor" for his defense of prepared breakfast cereals, failed to
mention was that mineral and trace element composition *is*
affected. And minerals like zinc are essential to health.

The adult daily allowance for zinc is 15 mg, and it is difficult
to get that much from food that has been processed or
carelessly cooked. Seafood, meat, and eggs are rich sources, as is
milk. Leafy green vegetables, nuts, and whole grains would be
good sources if the soil were not depleted of this vital nutrient.
Stress increases our need for zinc, and excess copper—either
from vitamin supplements or from copper pipes—drives out
zinc, as do the Pill and other medicines. Frozen green vegetables may be missing their natural component of zinc; it is also
removed from white flour.

Pill users need all the natural zinc they can get. Whenever
possible, they should use garden- or farm-fresh vegetables and
store them in the coldest spot possible. Buying small quantities
will avoid storage losses. For those foods which can't be eaten
raw, cooking should be slow, at low temperatures. All cooking
liquids should be used as part of the meal; the habit of adding
these liquids to a homemade soup is a healthy one, particularly
for Pill users.

Among the vegetables, peas and carrots are the best sources of zinc. Oysters, herring, and clams have a high content, but some of these seafoods come from contaminated water. Such seafood contains excess copper, which drives out the zinc. Whole wheat and oatmeal are excellent sources of zinc, and whole nuts and peanut butter are fair sources. The amount in these foods, however, depends upon the soil, and much of our soil is now zinc-poor.

Animal feeds are now enriched with zinc, and some of it gets passed on to us in animal foods. Cow's milk is a good source.

Vitamins C and E and the B complex seem to help zinc along. If it is taken as part of a vitamin therapy, 15 mg and certainly 30 mg will suffice for most conditions. Multivitamins usually contain too much copper and not enough zinc. Some health food stores stock zinc in 15 mg and 30 mg tablets; this dosage should not be exceeded once deficiencies have been corrected. Excess zinc may diminish selenium, which may have a protective effect against cancer. Too much zinc may also cause diarrhea, nausea, and vomiting.

Excesses of the Pill

For unknown reasons, the Pill produces excessive amounts of some nutrients in a woman's body. While many questions remain about these changes, Pill users should avoid supplements containing substantial amounts of copper, iron, niacin, and, sometimes, vitamin A.

Copper

Many Americans have too much copper in their diets, partly because of our use of copper water pipes. Depending upon the source of the water (acid well water tends to carry copper from the plumbing) and the condition of the pipes, a person may take in more than the RDA for copper with every glass of tap water. Copper sulfate is widely used today as a growth stimulant in meat animals, so copper gets served to us with our meat.

When zinc is deficient, the copper excess gets worse, and vice versa.

The Pill and other estrogens aggravate the zinc-copper imbalance. Dr. J. Cecil Smith, Jr., chief of the Trace Element Research Laboratory at the Washington, D.C., VA Hospital, studied a number of women who take the Pill. He found that those who suffered from Pill side effects showed a larger copper excess than those who had no symptoms.

Excess copper is particularly linked to iron-deficiency anemia, nausea, vomiting, and heart attacks. Copper may also increase blood clotting. It also acts as a stimulant to the brain and thus may contribute to the elevated blood pressure often found in women who take the Pill.

The excess-copper/low-zinc combination has also been associated with insomnia, depression, migraine, and hypomanic states similar to those produced by amphetamines. Migraines and other neurological disturbances in Pill users are viewed seriously, for they may precede strokes. After giving up the Pill, zinc supplements and the avoidance of excess copper are advisable.

Iron

Pill users show an increase in serum iron levels. The mechanism responsible for this change is unclear, since the reduction in menstrual flow is not large enough to account for the difference. The circulating iron, in tests so far, does not seem to deplete bone marrow, although the iron probably has been taken from the body's stores. Researchers now feel that the need for iron in Pill users is slightly decreased.

Vitamin A

Pill users show a significant increase in their serum vitamin A levels, generally 30 to 80 percent.

No one is quite sure where the A is coming from, or whether it will have untoward effects upon the woman. Since the measured increase is in the blood, researchers think that the vitamin is being stolen from the tissues. In theory, this leaves the woman with a vitamin A deficiency in the tissues and may leave her open to night blindness and lowered resistance to infections. Perhaps the fact that up to 40 percent of long-term Pill users become somewhat color-blind (they are particularly apt to have trouble distinguishing blue from yellow, according to Olaf Lagerlof, a Swedish eye specialist) is related to the contraceptive's peculiar interactions with vitamin A.

However, excessive A may lead to birth defects, so the former Pill user who wants a baby should avoid taking A to compensate for a "deficiency" that might not exist. If the excessive A is large enough, it is poisonous and may lead to death.

With all the uncertainty, it *is* known that vitamin A and estrogens are antagonistic. A is necessary to synthesize the hormone; but the hormone keeps the body from using A in a normal way. Changes in vitamin A metabolism are ominous enough to constitute sufficient reason for nutrition-conscious women to avoid the Pill.

For those who don't get enough A from their food—and the RDA for vitamin A is very large—the amount of A found in multivitamins (up to 5000 units) is probably acceptable, even with the Pill. But those who are getting enough dietary A and protein should avoid further supplements, particularly if they have symptoms of excess A. These include fatigue, insomnia, irritability, nerve lesions, hair loss, jaundice, itchy skin, loss of appetite, blood clotting changes, and painful bones and joints.

On stopping the Pill, some women develop extremely serious menorrhagia (heavy menstrual bleeding). In these cases they may be suffering a "rebound" effect of extremely low levels of bloodstream vitamin A. Should this condition occur (the vitamin A levels can be checked out in a laboratory), some nutritionists and doctors prescribe temporary megadoses of up to 60,000 units per day. This seems dangerously high, for vitamin A overdosage can be fatal, but more moderate supplements of 10,000 to 20,000 daily units sometimes suffice.

Foods that contain generous amounts of vitamin A include

most dark green and yellow-orange vegetables, including carrots, spinach, and parsley. Liver, liver oil, and halibut are also good sources.

Butter and cheese, with the exception of cottage cheese, include moderate amounts of vitamin A. Other foods containing A in moderate amounts include egg yolks, margarine, dried milk, cream, white fish, eel, kidneys (beef, pig, or lamb), liver (pork), mangoes, apricots, yellow melons, peaches, sour cherries, nectarines, beet greens, broccoli, endive, kale, mustard greens, pumpkin, sweet potatoes, watercress, tomatoes, leek greens, chicory, chives, collards, fennel, butterhead and romaine lettuce, chard, and winter squashes.

The Pill also interferes with other nutrients. While taking the Pill, a woman may need larger than normal amounts of B_1, B_2, and B_{12}, as well as moderate supplements of vitamin E (30 to 200 units) and perhaps a calcium and magnesium combination.

The basic regimen

Pill users, and those who are recovering from taking it, are very likely to need supplemental vitamins. Deficiencies vary from person to person, so the individual will have to adjust her therapy according to the response she gets.

We would suggest, as a start, this regimen:

1. High-potency therapeutic "stress formula" B complex with C, including folic acid and a minimum of 5 mg of B_6: one tablet twice daily.

* If depressed, failing to menstruate, or showing symptoms of diabetes, hypoglycemia, or severe premenstrual tension and bloating, add separately one 50 mg tablet of B_6 daily, or even two.

* If showing symptoms of bleeding gums, easy bruising, or spider veins, add one tablet of vitamin "C complex" containing the citrus bioflavonoids, hesperidin, and rutin; or else take a

daily bioflavonoid pill along with the normal stress-formula supplement.

2. One vitamin E plus selenium tablet (25 mcg selenium and 200 units of E) three times a week, or 100 to 200 units of E daily. If vitamin E cannot be taken after a meal with fats, lecithin should be swallowed with it.

3. Four hundred mcg of folic acid once a day if stress-formula supplement contains less than this amount.

4. Thirty to 50 mg of zinc three times a week if deficiency is suspected.

5. Ten thousand to 20,000 units of vitamin A daily *only if* menstrual bleeding is extremely heavy, if a "rebound" vitamin A deficiency has been established, and if conception is not planned.

Several single-pill vitamin supplements have been designed with the Pill user in mind, including the Pill Pill, Feminens, and Cefol. These supplements vary in the amounts of vitamin A, zinc, magnesium, folic acid, and other nutrients they contain. Care must be exercised to choose the correct vitamin pill, if the user is determined to have all her supplements in a single capsule.

We feel that the soundest approach to compensating for the Pill's nutritional effects is to take a good stress-formula supplement after breakfast and again after dinner. The combination of B complex and C, in divided doses, is a good basic regimen. Then the individual can add folic acid, B₆, E, bioflavonoids, and/or minerals, depending upon the deficiencies suspected. Vegetarians may benefit from additional B₁₂.

It may also be advisable to "vacation" from the vitamin regimen from time to time. Many people report that their vitamins work better if they stop taking them for a weekend or one weekend day. Others skip the vitamins for a few days to a week each month.

It does seem a shame to compensate for pills by taking more pills, even humble vitamins. The right supplements—in moderate doses, not megadoses—do relieve a number of the Pill's nuisance side effects and usually help the woman who is recovering from the Pill after quitting to get back to normal more rapidly. The reason for these improvements is well established—in nutrition and metabolism journals that few gynecologists ever see or read. With appropriate supplements, blood levels of the affected nutrients return to normal and deficiency symptoms are relieved. In some cases, such as folic-acid-deficiency anemia or severe B_6-depletion pharmacologic depression, vitamin supplements may actually save a Pill user's life.

Nonetheless, we suspect it may be unwholesome to mask the Pill's effects with further chemicals. Again, this is an example of biochemical roulette. For women who must stay on the Pill, even though they may be suffering, we have included the information in this chapter. We also feel that supplements are well worth taking for a few months to relieve the post-Pill syndrome, a condition little discussed by doctors but well known to women, who may feel terrible for an interim period after they stop the Pill. (They are undergoing withdrawal effects. Many of their normal processes have been disturbed and now require readjustment.)

Above all, Pill users should watch their diet, just as any sensible person should. They should study the basic food groups and make sure they get an ample natural supply of the nutrients apt to be depleted by the Pill. Unfortunately, there are Pill brand differences in how these nutrients may be affected, and these brand differences are only slightly understood. Any Pill user who cares about her long-term health and energy should learn about deficiency symptoms and watch for them in herself.† She should eat the foods that supply what her body seems to be lacking and, if she can afford it, she might wish to have her vitamin and mineral levels clinically tested.

† One of our other books, *Women and the Crisis in Sex Hormones* (Bantam, $3.50), includes vitamin tables that give more detailed information on deficiency symptoms and food groups that relieve them.

CHAPTER 15

There Are Better Ways: Alternatives to the Pill

At all ages, the lowest level of mortality by far is achieved
by a combined regimen, i.e., use of barrier contraceptives
with recourse to early abortion in case of failure.

> Christopher Tietze and Sarah Lewit
> The Population Council
> 1979

We have been led to think that birth control is a "modern miracle," but there were always some women, especially in the
upper classes, who had knowledge of effective contraceptive
techniques. Cleopatra, for example, used suppositories made
from dried crocodile dung (which is highly spermicidal) and
other ingredients in a honey base. Midwives and herbalists in
many cultures passed on their secret knowledge of plants and
teas, some of which, modern pharmacologists confirm, do have
contraceptive properties.

Then there was rhythm, or "organic" birth control. Calen-
dar-based rhythm is not too reliable, as few women enjoy clock-
work menstrual cycles. On the other hand, as women once
knew and are rediscovering, their bodies undergo many noticeable changes when ovulation is about to occur. Women who
train themselves in body awareness can feel slight ovulation
pain, which is technically known as mittelschmerz. The breasts

become more sensitive. There are measurable changes in the saliva, urine, vaginal secretions, and appearance of the cervix as the female body prepares itself for possible conception. We will return to these matters later, for, almost in secret, many women and couples are resuming organic birth control. Education and some further research are needed before these natural methods reach all of the potential users who might prefer them. The drug companies are opposed to them (no profits), while most doctors also minimize their value because it takes supervision out of their hands.

His responsibility or hers?

Margaret Sanger argued, with justice, that woman-controlled methods are an essential option, for some men will not or cannot take responsibility for their seed. She popularized the diaphragm, invented in the nineteenth century, and raised the research money to develop the Pill. Men who came of age in the Pill-and-IUD-dominated 1960s hardly knew that reliable methods existed for them. In fact, it had been male contraceptives—withdrawal and the condom—that drastically reduced the birthrate in modern times. Centuries before the crusades of Mrs. Sanger, such sexual sophisticates as Casanova not only advocated the condom (and the idea of male responsibility) but addressed their ingenuity to female methods, too. Casanova observed that a squeezed-out lemon half, placed over the cervix, provided both a mechanical barrier to sperm *and* a spermicide in the acidic lemon juice. Thus he discovered a precursor of the diaphragm and jelly, many years before they came into official use.

Carefully employed, the condom and even withdrawal are more effective than most people imagine (the condom is, like the IUD, a 97 percent effective method), but each has obvious drawbacks.*

Although it requires skill and discipline, withdrawal was the

---

* A 97 percent method means that if one hundred couples use that method for one year, three pregnancies will result.

sole method of contraception used by two thirds of the couples in France and Hungary until 1960! The birthrate in these countries was admirably low. It shouldn't be overlooked as a method for emergencies.

Condoms

But it is the humble condom, which, like the lead pencil, the bicycle, and the razor blade, more than holds its own today in a sea of technological wonders. Worldwide, the condom, or sheath, is still the number one method of birth control, the preferred method in such sexually sophisticated, low-birthrate nations as Japan, England, and Sweden.

The clever Japanese make a condom one-third to one-half as thick as ours (but equally reliable) and provide it in unusual colors and a variety of shapes that heighten their erotic pleasure. The Swedes, conscious of its efficiency at preventing the spread of disease, stopped a galloping VD epidemic in its tracks by their successful promotion of the condom. In the United States we are reluctant to sell teenagers on the condom's advantages and ban it from being advertised on TV. We seem to prefer that our young people get infected first—then we'll tell them on the air where to find a clinic to treat the disease. In fact, contrary to general belief, in many communities high school boys still have difficulty buying condoms, as druggists may refuse to sell to minors.

U.S.-made condoms must meet rigorous federal standards. They are tested electronically for pinholes by the manufacturer, for burst and tensile strength, and are guaranteed to have a shelf life of at least two years. The thickness of American condoms ranges from 1.05 to 1.09 mm, and unlike the makers of some foreign versions, which come in small, medium, and large, American manufacturers assume that "one size fits all." This theory is no truer for condoms than it is for, say, women's panty hose. There are always persons at either end of the scale who are poorly fitted. The condom companies could go all out and give their sizes fancy, macho names, the equivalent of "Ferrari," "Jaguar," and "Rolls-Royce." Or perhaps take a tip from the olive companies and size their products "jumbo," "colossal," and "super-colossal." Not only comfort but reliability is at stake. Just as average-size condoms slip off men in the smaller range, they break when the user is extra well endowed. If condoms *were* available in a range of sizes, they might well become a 99 percent method, like the diaphragm or the Pill.

Condoms are available dry or lubricated. Most users prefer lubricated brands, for lubrication facilitates entry, decreases chances of breaking, and increases sensitivity. A dry or "silicone" lubricant is preferred by many, for it is odorless and provides a slippery surface rather than a wet one.

There are several variations in condom shape, which have long been popular in the Orient but are newer to the United States. Preshaped condoms may reduce the chance of slipping and are also preferred by some as being more sensitive. Transparent condoms are generally, but not always, preferred to opaque, and the colors now available appeal to a wide spectrum of users.

When condoms are not hermetically sealed, there is an increased chance that dirt or other particles may damage the latex, especially if the contraceptives are carried around in wallets. It is therefore important for reliability that the condom selected be hermetically sealed.

A condom should be placed on the erect penis before penetration, as many men, when sexually aroused, secrete several drops of precoital fluid that occasionally contain enough live sperm to cause fertilization. If the condom lacks a reservoir tip, space should be left at the end to catch the discharge. If a dry condom is selected, lubrication of the outside with a spermicidal cream or jelly prevents tearing and facilitates entry, but petroleum jelly is not recommended because it can cause the rubber to deteriorate.

Men who don't like condoms say they interfere with sensation. They might try the more expensive versions derived from animal membranes, rather than latex, as the lubricants used to make so-called skin condoms cling to the penis create temperature changes on evaporation that may enhance the wearer's pleasure. They might also look into the latex brands specially formulated to provide extra friction (Excita by Schmid is one example) and thus particularly appreciated by some women. In Japan it is customary for women to put the condom in place as part of foreplay.

To summarize the art of choosing condoms: get them in the Orient if you can. Japanese condoms made for import to the United States must still meet the arbitrary thickness requirements our government has set. Nonetheless, the new American condoms have advantages that make some brands acceptable, even enjoyable, to some men and enhance the pleasure of some women. Though many users prefer more expensive models, lubrication is the most critical issue, and here price is not a significant factor. Nor is price a factor in selecting for reliability where it is a question of checking that the package is hermetically sealed.

Heat

Heat, X ray, diathermy, and laser beams may also temporarily or permanently inhibit the production of sperm and are being investigated as methods of contraception. There is little question that heat, including fever, reduces fertility some of the time. Today the first thing many infertility specialists tell their male patients is to stop wearing tight jockey shorts or trousers, which, by maintaining the scrotum too close to the body, temporarily sterilize some men.

TMS (standing for thermatic method of Temporary Male Sterilization) as developed by Martha Voegeli, a Swiss doctor, in India, works like this: for three weeks a man takes a daily forty-five-minute bath in water of 116 degrees Fahrenheit. This procedure should render him sterile for six months, after which his normal fertility returns. A man wishing to try this method should get a sperm count following the three-week treatment to make sure he has achieved the wanted result. Were simple sperm-count tests for home use to be developed, TMS might even become a popular contraceptive option.

Sterilization for men

The male vas deferens is handily located outside the main body, and so, since the abdomen need not be entered, vasectomy is not considered major surgery. The operation prevents the sperm from getting into the semen by cutting or blocking the tubes that carry it from the testicles to the penis. Ejaculation continues as usual, although the seminal fluid cannot fertilize. Sexual sensations normally remain unaltered.

No vasectomy deaths have been reported in the United States in many years. Nonetheless, the procedure requires a skilled surgeon. And there can be side effects, too. About half of the men who have the operation may get some skin discoloration and swelling (both are harmless and disappear after a few weeks), and some pain either when the anesthetic is injected or, more commonly, during intercourse for a time following the procedure.

Both superficial and deep infections are possible, but most will respond well to antibiotics. Swelling and tenderness may be treated with drugs, bed rest, heat, and the wearing of a suspensory.

Studies show that it does no damage to a man's general health, although theoretical questions have been raised about the long-term effect of a vasectomy on autoimmune responses. One half or more vasectomized males develop an immunity to sperm within their own body, and some scientists fear the reaction may predispose to a class of illnesses called collagen diseases, which include rheumatoid arthritis, in later life. No evidence has yet been found to support this concern. Probably the antibodies serve simply to destroy the unreleased sperm.

Two well-known men who have broadcast their satisfaction with vasectomy are Arthur Godfrey and Jim Bouton. They stress the peace of mind the operation brings. When Bouton told Germaine Greer about his operation, on a TV talk show, she declared, "That's the sexiest thing a man has said to me in a long time."

But Godfrey and Bouton also point out that vasectomy will not cure a bad marriage or potency problems. Sometimes, when men doubt their masculinity, vasectomy makes matters worse.

John Gagnon, a former Kinsey Institute researcher, suggests that any man contemplating sterilization should ask himself these questions: Do I want more children? If my children died, would I want to replace them? Were I as rich as, say, the Kennedys, then would I want more children? If I broke up with my wife and she got custody, would I want more children of my own? Does the image of a knife being taken to my testicles give me the creeps?

Gagnon, who had a vasectomy about fifteen years ago, satisfied himself that his personal answer to all these questions was no.

While some vasectomies (no more than a quarter) can be surgically reversed, a man should never count on reversal, nor on the possibility that his sperm might be frozen and used later on. For unexplained reasons, the semen of breed bulls and other animals can be more successfully preserved than human sperm. An important area of birth control research would, we think, be the perfection of sperm banks. When this occurs, vasectomy will become attractive to a larger number of men, even perhaps teenagers.

Many surgeons believe they need to "interview" vasectomy prospects in order to ensure that their motivations are sound. Counseling is extremely useful for the undecided, and full disclosure of possible complications is essential, but we maintain that only the patient can make the ultimate decision. Indeed, the man should interview the surgeon, whose services he is *buying*, to ensure that the doctor is highly experienced.

On occasion, the surgeon forgets to explain that vasectomy does not render that patient sterile at once. It takes a number of ejaculations and the passage of time (weeks or months) before the sperm already in the semen is cleared. The man must

return for sperm counts and continue other birth control in the
meanwhile.

Temporary vasectomies—the insertion of plugs and valves instead of cutting—have been much touted by hopeful inventors.
Be wary of these experimental procedures, for the reversal rate
is hardly satisfactory. A narrow, living channel like the vas tends
to scar over when a foreign body is inserted. Many researchers
doubt that temporary vasectomy will ever become a reality.

The Pill for men

In the search for a male Pill, scientists have chiefly tried variations on the female version, using synthetic hormones to fool
the pituitary into diminishing its FSH and LH (stimulants to
the reproductive cells), and thus turn off production of sperm
in the gonads (as the female Pill inhibits release of the ova).
Any contraceptive that works through pituitary suppression is
bound to have some long-range effects on the entire body, of
which the pituitary is deemed the master gland. At best, male
contraceptives based on hormones are unlikely to be safer than
the current female Pills. They can be justified, perhaps, only on
the basis that they will provide a fine Sincerity Test for men
who claim they would die for love.

Though no male Pill has been approved and marketed as
such, one does exist and is on the shelf of every drugstore. Li-
censed by the FDA for the treatment of osteoporosis (bone
loss) and "male menopause," it has been shown to prevent
sperm production in young volunteers. Using such a product
for a purpose for which it was not designed would be like the
athletes' use of anabolic steroids (approved by the FDA for pituitary dwarfism, some anemias, and a few conditions of old
age) to build their bodies. But as one sports reporter at the
1976 Olympics noted, correctly, "The Breakfast of Champions
ain't Wheaties."

The secretly available male Pill—there are several brands—
contains large amounts of testosterone and a dollop of estrogen. The effects appear reversible after stopping. While we

don't advocate hormones for any healthy person (when a clock is working, you don't tinker with it), we acknowledge that for couples who feel they must use hormonal birth control it might be more sporting to pool the risks. She could take her Pill for a year and then rest her body while he has his turn.

There is also some research into male contraceptives not involving hormones or pituitary suppression. Drugs are being sought, for example, that work only locally on the epididymis, a part of the sperm transport mechanism. Should these materialize, they could, in theory, be far safer than hormones.

Many drugs inhibit sperm formation in the testes, or, if you prefer, testicles (the words are synonymous), without interfering with natural hormones. Thus far, all have exhibited unacceptable side effects, but the search goes on. One group, the nitrofurans, has had wide use as inhibitors of bacterial growth, but dosages high enough to sterilize are extremely toxic. Other sperm suppressants are found among cancer drugs and (at least in mice) in a sugar analogue.

In breakthrough research conducted in New Orleans, Andrew Schally recently isolated the hypothalamic chemicals that trigger the release of LH and FSH from the pituitary. Based on his discoveries, scientists in many laboratories are now seeking hypothalamic sperm suppressants, but there is some indication that they may diminish libido.

The Chinese Pill

In November 1978 a group from the Planned Parenthood Federation of America who were touring China made a startling discovery. The Chinese have a Pill for men! The drug is a well-known chemical made from cottonseed that is used here in the rubber industry. Sex drive is not affected, Chinese scientists say, and neither is subsequent fertility. American researchers are skeptical, but tests at New York City's Rockefeller University have been announced. It may not be coincidental that in China almost half of the doctors are women, whereas our contraceptive researchers are predominantly male.

The IUD

Another popular though risky method of birth control for women is the IUD, or intrauterine device. According to Food and Drug Administration figures, it is as likely as the Pill to land a woman in the hospital, though less likely to land her in the morgue. Few people know that with careful use the condom and foam are each as reliable as the IUD, and much safer.

The IUD is a device, nowadays most often made of copper, placed by the physician in the woman's uterus. Women who are older and who have had children are usually most comfortable with it. Though in a single year there have been no more than thirty-nine deaths attributed to the IUD, the wearer risks anemia, perforations, longer and more painful periods, severe pelvic infection, and hysterectomy.

And if she does get pregnant, it's a medical emergency if the IUD is still in place. Perforations are also medical emergencies. They occur when the IUD makes its way through the wall of the uterus into the abdomen. One can get a serious infection just from having an IUD inserted, and gonorrhea as well as staph and strep infections are a grave risk to the IUD wearer, for the exquisitely painful PID (pelvic inflammatory disease) that can develop often renders women permanently sterile.

IUD's are particularly hazardous to insert following childbirth or a miscarrage or abortion. At this time the expulsion rate—loss of the IUD—is more than one in four, and the patient may not be aware that she is unprotected. Perforations are also more apt to occur as the uterus involutes, or returns to normal size, a process that takes up to six or eight weeks. The safest time to insert an IUD is during normal menstruation. Anyone with anemia is advised against these devices because they usually cause extra bleeding and longer periods. Fibroids, endometriosis (a disorder of the endometrial tissue in the uterus), a small uterus, and heart disease are other contraindications. No one with any active infection should get one, and some researchers believe IUD's can reactivate past cases of gonorrhea. And no one, we think, should wear an IUD for more than five years because of the chronic inflammation it causes in the uterus, as well as the permanent damage—ridges and indentations—it produces in the uterine wall.

Since 1979 the FDA has required doctors to give every IUD patient a long, printed warning. Many doctors have not complied. If you, or a friend, have an IUD or are thinking of getting one, demand the warning and study it with care. You may change your mind.

Excessive bleeding can sometimes be controlled with vitamin C and bioflavonoids (known as the "capillary" factors, the bioflavonoids occur with C in nature, as in the pulpy portions of citrus fruit). Cramps may be reduced by calcium or calcium-magnesium pills, along with vitamin D. (See Chapter 14.)

Many people know that the Dalkon Shield is treacherous, but other models are proving equally so. Partly because its manufacturer, A. H. Robins, was honest in reporting complications, the Dalkon Shield is just the Lieutenant Calley of IUD's.

If possible, do not have an IUD inserted on a first visit to a doctor or clinic. First get a thorough examination, including VD and pregnancy tests, as well as an exploration of the physical condition of your uterus. Ask for a copy of the FDA-mandated warning and take it home with you to study. Probably, before getting an IUD, you should be checked for anemia too. The chances are no more than fifty-fifty that you will turn out to be a suitable candidate for the IUD. Should you have a uterine condition or an infection that would preclude it, it is far safer to find out before the insertion.

At the University of Texas in Houston, Dr. Waldemar Schmidt, a pathologist, has recently advised that intrauterine devices always be replaced at two-year intervals. He has discovered a new culprit in IUD infections. The vaginal flora changes in IUD wearers, according to Dr. Schmidt. Calcium deposits may encrust over the IUD in time, and these interact with actinomyces bacteria, producing explosive and sudden infections.

Schmidt cites a recent study by the Center for Disease Control in Atlanta, showing that 8 percent of IUD users show actinomyces on Pap tests. Serious infections are most apt to erupt in "precisely those women most comfortable with their IUD's —who have no cramping, spotting, or heavy periods and so go on wearing them for years." Most of the affected women are in their twenties and thirties, have had their IUD's in place for around six years, and have then developed clinical signs such as mild pain in the lower abdomen, cervical discharge, fever, and chills. Some have night sweats, menstrual irregularity, and weight loss.

To avoid surgery and ultimate sterility, it is crucial to have a culture taken at the first indication of an IUD infection. Different "bugs" are responsive to different antibiotic treatments, and many doctors get poor results because they are not specific enough in selecting the medication.

Some cautious students of IUD's feel that no woman who has ever had gonorrhea, or other sexually transmitted infections, should take her chance with this birth control device. It appears that in some cases an old and presumably cured infection is made to flare up again by insertion of an IUD.

The diaphragm

Of all the methods a woman can initiate, the diaphragm and cervical cap are the most effective alternatives to the Pill. In some ways these methods are better than the Pill, for the woman controls them more if she is conscientious. In actual use the Pill is not quite the 99 percent effective method manufacturers boast of. A national fertility survey showed that during the first year they took it, 6 percent of Pill users got pregnant. After that the figure declined. Doctors and manufacturers used to blame these "breakthrough" pregnancies on missed pills, but there is recent evidence that certain common drugs sometimes block the contraceptive action of the Pill. These include some antihistamines, barbiturates, and other drugs: specifically, Amytal, Nembutal, phenobarbital, Seconal, Butazolidin, Dilantin, Equanil, Miltown, Rimactane.

Backed up by legal abortion in those rare cases of failure, the motivated woman can feel safe and not sorry, protected by the diaphragm, the same old "rubber parachute" that helped her mother keep a family down to size. Women—and men—are newly aware of the diaphragm's efficiency and the safety record of abortions. But many still trust the diaphragm too little and the Pill and the IUD too much.

A study reported in 1976 by the Sanger Research Bureau— the largest ever done on contemporary U.S. diaphragm users— has shown the diaphragm to be highly reliable even when used by young single women and teenagers. It rates better than most IUD's and also the minipill (progestin-only pill). Of the 2,168 women covered by the Sanger study, only 37, or 2 percent, had accidental pregnancies. Of these, 22 admitted that "they had used the diaphragm inconsistently or not at all." The study revealed that the diaphragm is better than 99 percent reliable for those who use it faithfully.

The Sanger study surprised a lot of people who had thought that the final word from Masters and Johnson was that you couldn't trust the diaphragm. Masters and Johnson had reported that when a woman is sexually excited, the inner portion of her vaginal canal expands and her diaphragm may no longer fit well. If at that moment the penis escapes the vagina and is reinserted, it may displace the diaphragm or even enter the "danger zone" between the rim of the device and the wall of the vagina.

But the Sanger study showed that even when a woman might be exposed because of the "loss of correct diaphragm positioning during the excitement and plateau stages of sexual response," she was in fact protected. Apparently the spermicidal cream or jelly used with the diaphragm provides the extra insurance.

A diaphragm costs about six dollars and must be carefully fitted by a doctor, nurse, or paramedic, and the person being fitted should know of the various models available and be sure she had been offered the most comfortable choice for her. The ideal diaphragm can be found for almost every woman, but the patient must participate in the selection. Moreover, she must find a doctor or technician who knows the diaphragm's value—some doctors trained in the sixties do not, and are not skilled in fitting it. Others resent the amount of time it takes to instruct the patient thoroughly. The best choice is the doctor or technician who boasts, "My diaphragm patients never get pregnant," and who will take an hour or more to coach a first-time user. Fitting fees start at around fifteen dollars in private offices, but may be less at clinics. A woman may need a larger size after childbirth, abortion, or pelvic surgery and in any case should have the device checked about once a year. Since doctors deem their time so precious, diaphragm fitting is not cost-effective. Nurses and paramedics often do a better job. If a diaphragm hurts, it's not properly fitted.

The spermicidal creams and jellies used with the diaphragm sell for four or five dollars for a tube good for a dozen applications. One teaspoonful is liberally applied on the inner side of the diaphragm and more is spread around the rim. Some women prefer spreading the jelly thinly on both sides of the diaphragm. The best protection results from using a stronger jelly or cream sold as a contraceptive on its own, not one designed to be used with diaphragms.

The Sanger clinic recommends that the diaphragm with the spermicide be put in place as much as six hours before it is needed, and left undisturbed for a minimum of six hours after intercourse. This recommendation appeals to women who think it unromantic to stop making love for the humdrum reason of self-protection. However, growing numbers of men in the United States have learned to assist with diaphragm insertion and include it as part of the foreplay.

If a woman expects a second sex encounter more than six hours after the first, she may prefer to remove the diaphragm, wash it and herself, reapply the jelly, and reinsert the diaphragm. If, however, second and third encounters occur soon after the first, the original spermicide is probably still active. Nonetheless, it is wise to add some extra jelly or cream, which can be purchased in prefilled disposable applicators. If more than six hours have passed and she hasn't removed her diaphragm, the back-up spermicide is essential.

And yet some women who don't like using these chemicals ("greasy kid stuff," they were called by 1960s-style swingers) have confided to us that for them the diaphragm alone works just fine. All diaphragms do not shift during sexual excitement. Half stay in place, and by trial and error certain women have learned that they are in this fortunate category.

It isn't known yet whether this depends on personal anatomy, fit, or the type of diaphragm selected, but inexpensive research (which isn't being done) could probably clarify which women, or which diaphragms, do not require spermicides. Such knowledge would make the diaphragm a far more convenient and economical option. So would clarification of which spermicides have the longest-acting base materials, for some, it is rumored, are good for twenty hours.

A woman inserts a diaphragm while sitting on the edge of a chair, lying flat on her back with knees bent, squatting, or propping up one leg on the seat of a chair. First she treats it with fresh spermicidal cream or jelly, then pinches it together and inserts it into the vagina as far as it will go, pressing the forward rim behind the ridge of the pubic bone. She removes it by hooking her finger behind the nearer rim and pulling downward. Then she washes it in mild soap and warm water, dusts it with cornstarch, and puts it away. And each time before she uses it, she first holds it up to the light to be sure it is still sound—that no holes have developed.

The cervical cap

There is another equally harmless and reliable barrier device that many women prefer to the diaphragm. The only difficulty is that the device is very hard to find in the United States, though available in some European countries.

A cervical cap looks something like a thimble. Made of rubber, lucite, or polyethylene, it fits over the cervix (the neck of the womb that juts into the vagina) and can be left undisturbed except during menstruation. It stays put by suction and is thought by some experts to require no jelly or cream, though they can be used.

Putting on a cap has been described as no harder than slipping a thimble on your finger in the dark—once you're accustomed to it. Many women use a little spermicidal cream or jelly for extra protection. A few men say that they feel the cap during intercourse, especially one made of a hard material such as lucite. Some women, on the other hand, claim the cap enhances their sexual response. Its beauty is that, just like the diaphragm, it can be inserted only when needed, or it can be worn continuously throughout the month, being removed only when a woman menstruates. It's probably healthiest to remove the cap periodically, at least when bathing or showering, to avoid any discharge or irritation. A woman squats or half lies down to insert her cap and leaves it in for at least six to eight hours following intercourse.

Two U.S. companies used to make the cap, but discontinued it because it's such a low-profit item. (The profit in diaphragms is mainly from accompanying spermicides. Also, the cap lasts longer.) At Chicago Lying-In Hospital and at the Albert Einstein Medical Center in New York City, researchers are trying to develop semipermanent caps, like dental bridges, with a valve for the discharge of menstrual flow. (Indeed, one of the researchers, Dr. Robert Goepp of Chicago, *is* a dentist, which is how he got the idea.)

Most authorities who are interested in *healthy* contraception fear that semipermanent caps, while less injurious than the IUD, might not be as benign as the removable models. On the other hand, the cap designed by Dr. Goepp and his colleague Uwe Freese, a gynecologist, has started to arouse widespread support and interest and was recently praised in a *Journal of the American Medical Association* editorial. Unfortunately, it is not yet commercially available, although it is undergoing clinical trials.

Members of the National Women's Health Network and self-help clinics have started to import caps from England, after failing to convince U.S. manufacturers to resume production.

In 1978 and 1979 the English caps became quite popular at some women-run clinics and even with a few physicians. Then, in a surprising move, the FDA began seizing shipments and attempted to ban the cap's use as a contraceptive in this country. With support from Dr. Philip Corfman, chief of the government's Contraceptive Research Branch, the National Women's Health Network led a battle to remove the ban. On behalf of the Network, this author testified at hearings on women's health care conducted by Senator Edward Kennedy in August 1979. It is my belief, as I stated at the hearings, that the ban was attempted for reasons of greed. Pharmaceutical companies dislike the cap because they fear it may cut into spermicide sales. Some physicians feel threatened by the impending popularity of the cap. It takes more time to teach a beginner than they like to spend. In some areas, such as New Hampshire, where nurses and paramedics are allowed to provide barrier birth control, use of the cap has been growing at a rapid pace, taking away clients from the doctors.

For the time being, the ban has been lifted and import from England continues. Dr. Corfman is supporting studies to determine the cap's precise effectiveness and ideal use. (Earlier studies, mostly performed in Europe, indicate that it is at least as reliable as the diaphragm.)

Interested clinics and physicians can order the cap from:

> Lamberts Ltd.
> 200 Queensbridge Road
> Dalston, London E.8
> England

In Brookline, Massachusetts, Dr. James Koch, with the help of several well-trained assistants, has fitted more than 1,100 caps. He has kept up-to-date lists of U.S. physicians and clinics who have caps available. For information, send him a stamped, self-addressed envelope:

> James Koch, M.D.
> 1037 Beacon Street
> Brookline, Mass. 02146

For $2.00, the National Women's Health Network also has a packet of cervical cap information, along with a current list of United States providers, which was compiled by Karel Joyce Littman. The address is:

> National Women's Health Network
> 224 Seventh Street, S.E.
> Washington, D.C. 20003

Personnel at the New Hampshire Feminist Health Center, who were among the very first in the United States to revive the cap, have trained other providers, including nurses, lay health workers, and physicians, in its proper use. The center also has an information packet, which is updated continuously. It costs $5.00. Write to:

> New Hampshire Feminist Health Center
> 38 South Main Street
> Concord, N.H. 03301

Perhaps because of anatomical variations, the current models of cervical cap cannot be fitted to every woman. At present, according to reports from clinics and from physicians such as Dr. Koch, about three women in four can be satisfactorily fitted. Dr. Koch and others are researching new designs.

Specific Instructions for Use: At most of the women-run clinics, patients are instructed to remove their cap daily for caution's sake. Before each new insertion, a dollop of spermicide is usually added. Even with this regimen, the cap, unlike the diaphragm, can be completely separated from lovemaking, forgotten for a day at a time. Dr. Koch, on the other hand, instructs his patients to leave their caps in place for three days, then five, and then even a week if they still find spermicide remaining when they take it out. Among the brands of spermicide being used with the cap are Delfen Cream, Ramses 5 percent Nonoxynol Jelly, and Koromex Cream II. When the latter is used, Dr. Koch recommends reducing the maximum number of days between removals to three or four. In his research, Dr. Koch is attempting to establish precisely which brands of spermicide remain active within the cap for the longest period of time.

When caps are left in on a weekly schedule, they may develop an unpleasant odor. In fact, Dr. Koch reports that this is the most frequent side effect or complaint he has thus far encountered. To overcome this problem, the caps can be soaked for twelve hours in rubbing alcohol or in water mixed with either chlorophyll or a product called Nilodor, available in drugstores. Some women prefer to mix a few drops of chlorophyll with their spermicide before inserting the cap. Others let the cap soak, for about twenty minutes, in a cup of water to which a tablespoon of cider vinegar or lemon juice has been added.

Teenagers

Strongly as we recommend the diaphragm for many women, it is not always the ideal solution for the teenaged sexual initiate—or anyone who has been chaste for several years or longer —as her size may alter in the first few months of sexual activity. Nor, for health reasons, are the Pill and IUD advisable, for the very young. Moreover, sexually active kids need to protect themselves from VD as well as pregnancy. Yet most kids don't think of going to a clinic for birth control information until they're in trouble, a recent study from Johns Hopkins shows.

We feel the best answer for the young girl is spermicidal foam and a boyfriend with a condom. Common spermicidal creams and foams are powerful killers of syphilis and gonorrhea organisms, as well as nearly thirty other infections transmitted through sexual contact, including herpes. In a more realistic world, both foam and condoms would be freely available in drugstores as well as in rest-room vending machines, but they are still under-the-counter items in many states. And as a television writer discovered when his adolescent love scene for a popular show was altered, the current level of public morality is that sex between teenagers is okay on the airways as long as the youngsters worry a lot afterward.

Among spermicides for solo use (as distinguished from those

made to be spread on the diaphragm or squeezed into the cap), aerosol foams are the most reliable and easiest to use. Foam distributes immediately, while cream or jellies take several minutes. Both offer protection for several hours. Suppositories may deliver the least effective distribution. Some consider foam costly, as it averages 35 to 40 cents per application—more if the woman uses a double dose. But it's like a fire extinguisher: you pay only when you are in need, so it's not too bad a bargain.

In 1974 a study by Dr. Gerald Bernstein of 3,000 Los Angeles women, mostly from poor neighborhoods, indicated the surprising reliability of foam. Of the women who completed the study, the pregnancy rate in one year for women using foam alone was 4 per 100 women, a remarkably low rate for clinic patients with demanding mates and chaotic lives.

The patients had been trained in the correct use of foam by neighborhood paramedics who spoke their own language. In earlier clinic studies that showed lower reliability, many of the women had douched out the foam, or used it *after* having sex relations.

Couples past forty find foam almost as successful as the Pill, and far less dangerous—1 percent failure rate for the Pill, 2 for foam. By 1970 as many women were using foam as the IUD and, when they used it conscientiously, achieved excellent results. An underground of women physicians, health workers, and doctors' wives were using it but didn't say so in public until the Bernstein study showed it wasn't a fluke.

Foam should be inserted no more than an hour before intercourse. Nor need it inhibit oral sex. Since it is as easy to put in as a tampon, a woman can wait to apply it until the moment just before actual intercourse.

Half of the women who try foam find it messy. A few find it irritating, or their lovers do, but a simple brand switch often resolves the latter problem. For those who do like the texture, especially women with poor lubrication, foam is an excellent method, which has probably been downgraded by the medical profession because it's not doctor-controlled. When a double dose is employed, foam may be on a par with the diaphragm and Pill, 99 percent reliable. Combined with the condom, it gives the most absolute protection available.

Spermicidal suppositories

The newer versions, with names such as Encare and Intercept, are being heavily promoted and advertised. The manufacturers imply or claim that they are 99 percent reliable, or better than foam. FDA is presently checking whether the claims are legitimate, but, for the meantime, it is probably safest to assume that foam and condoms remain the most reliable over-the-counter methods. Suppositories may produce a tingling or burning sensation as they dissolve. Some women find it mildly pleasant, while others complain that it is quite uncomfortable.

Organic birth control: working with nature

If women all shared the same menstrual patterns, or had cycles of the same length, the calendar method of birth control could be the answer, for it's not hard to calculate the safe days before ovulation, the fertile days, and then the safe days after. But most women's cycles vary by an average of seven to thirteen days in the span of a year, if they are in their twenties and thirties, and by far greater amounts as teenagers, or when approaching menopause.

To use the calendar method, a woman records her menstrual history for six to twelve months to determine how many days there are between her periods. She can assume she will ovulate fourteen or fifteen days before she begins to menstruate, so if her cycles seem exceptionally regular, she need abstain from intercourse for only six days—three days before her assumed ovulation and three after.

But in the space of a year only 5 to 15 percent of women remain that regular. To be at all safe, most must assume a nine-day fertile period, from the tenth through the eighteenth days of the cycle, which means a woman must avoid sex for almost a third of her procreative life. It's asking a lot of her and her partner. Nonetheless, the rhythm method was popular until about 1960, when the women practicing it started switching to the Pill. By 1970 the number of American women following the method had dropped from 20 percent to 5 percent.

There are other ways to find out which are the fertile days, and one is the temperature method. A woman's basal body temperature (taken with an oral or rectal thermometer at the very start of the day, before eating, drinking, smoking, or conversation) rises in the latter part of her cycle as an effect of the progesterone increase that accompanies the release of the egg; the rise is about 0.5 to 1.0 degrees Fahrenheit. By avoiding intercourse until three days *after* the rise, and allowing it only in the remaining days before menstruation, most women can reliably prevent conception. But they also reduce their active sex lives even more. Some experienced women combine calendar and temperature methods to find the moment of ovulation more precisely, so they can more safely reduce their days of abstention to the basic six.

There are other signals in her body besides temperature that a woman can learn to interpret to discover which part of her cycle she's in, and those who have done so are making this a new era of natural birth control. One element in her body that goes through obvious changes is her cervical mucus. After menstruation there is a phase when there is only a little discharge, sometimes a sensation of dryness. Then the mucus becomes thick and sticky. At mid-cycle, when she ovulates, the discharge increases in volume, becoming clear and highly lubricative, with the consistency of egg white. At the end of the cycle the mucus may assume any of various patterns, but is no longer stretchy, like a raw egg. It is during the preovulation and mid-cycle phase, and just after, that a woman must abstain from unprotected sex.

The trouble with tracking one's cycle by checking mucus is that only 70 percent of women can do it with confidence. Others can't find a discernible pattern. Moreover, the method requires discipline on the part of both woman and man. Some couples learn to substitute noncoital methods of satisfaction, such as oral sex, during mid-cycle.

Mucus readings should be taken late in the day. And as with other rhythm methods, the average period of abstinence is pretty long—ten days out of a twenty-eight-day cycle. Some modern couples find that if the man as well as the woman takes part in the mucus checking and chart keeping, the method is more successful. One teacher also points out there's no reason the couple couldn't use the condom during this ten-day period. If a diaphragm was used, she says, the spermicides might make it harder to determine the state of the cervical mucus. An excellent guidebook for women who wish to master ovulation timing is Nora Aguilar's *No-Pill No-risk Birth Control* (New York: Rawson, Wade, 1980).

To help the 30 percent who can't do it themselves, even with the assistance of their partner, a way has been invented to show them what their body mucus is saying. Harold Kosasky, a fertility specialist from Boston, has created a device he calls an Ovutimer, into which a woman can insert samples of her cervical mucus each day. The Ovutimer measures the thickness of the mucus, and the arm of the device drops when the woman is close to ovulation. The Ovutimer is now being tested as a contraceptive (it was created to help women who want to conceive), and its inventor claims it works so well most women need be abstinent only sixty hours. Kosasky's patients have had excellent results with it. He hopes an inexpensive home model will be available soon.

Kosasky claims that the only women who will not be able to use an Ovutimer are those with abnormal cervical mucus, caused by infection (such as VD), by certain rare disease, or by taking hormones (such as the Pill). Even women with longer than usual fertility periods don't confound the Ovutimer. They, too, can be sure, when the arm of the Ovutimer has stopped dropping, that they can soon relax and have sex without worry.

Still another variant on the rhythm method was worked out by Louise Lacey, author of *Lunaception,* and is based on the findings of a physicist, Edmund Dewan. Lacey's method depends on regulating her periods by sleeping with the light on in her bedroom during the fourteenth through sixteenth nights of her cycle. Since 1972 Lacey has used no means of contraception except abstention from sex during her period of ovulation, which she can now control through the manipulation of light.

Feminist health workers have developed yet another way to determine a woman's unsafe, or fertile, period by observing the changes not in her mucus but in her cervix. With this method, a woman inserts a speculum in her own vagina and reads the changes with the help of a mirror and a strong light source. The cervix is tight and firm at the outset, becomes loose and droopy, then soft and moist. It is also light pink at ovulation, and dark pink as menstruation approaches.

Another "organic" method is being investigated by researchers Gerald and Selmaree Oster, who are tracking the chemical changes in saliva and urine over the course of the monthly cycle.

Their tests detect the surge of LH—the pituitary hormone that marks the second half of the cycle—and their goal is that a woman should, say, be able to apply a "matchstick" to the tip of her tongue; this "matchstick" would then turn red, signaling "Stop," when ovulation approaches.

Another chemist, Dr. George Preti of the Monell Chemical Senses Center, University of Pennsylvania, has been examining vaginal and mouth secretions for the occurrence of lactic acid and other components that evidence a cyclical rise and fall. Preti has received a substantial grant from the United States Department of Agriculture so that his findings might be applied to improve artificial insemination techniques in cattle. He has not been able to get support for continuing his human studies, even though, like the Osters', his work has the potential for evolving into a "matchstick" ovulation test.

Sterilization for women

For men or women, sterilization is a serious decision. In women it involves cutting, blocking, crushing, or cauterizing both Fallopian tubes. Female sterilization is always major surgery even when deceptively simple terms like "belly button" or "Band-Aid procedure" are used to "sell" it. The mortality rate ranges from 20 to 30 per 100,000. The operation requires a skilled surgeon, and there may be unexpected consequences. Five percent have serious complications, which include cardiac arrest, hemorrhage, severe infection, perforation or burning of the intestines, and pulmonary embolism. Some women develop periods of depression; others, a striking increase in menstrual complaints. Fifteen percent say they regret the surgery, while two thirds of the rest are only "moderately" satisfied.

Nonetheless, sterilization of one or the other partner has become the most popular form of birth control for American couples past thirty, and surprisingly, more women than men are having the operation, despite the much graver risks. Female sterilization is almost never reversible. However, as most people are surprised to learn, sterilization is *not* a 100 percent method. Occasionally, in women and in men, the severed tubes rejoin as part of a long-term healing process. When this happens to a man the harm he suffers is unexpected paternity. (In Pennsylvania, one such fellow tried to sue his surgeon and lost: the judge ruled that the birth of a healthy infant is no grounds for collecting damages.)

When it happens to a woman, the story is entirely different. Usually her tubes have healed sufficiently for sperm to meet egg, but not enough to allow passage of the conceptus into the uterus. Ectopic pregnancy, a life-threatening emergency, results.

Young or single white women may have difficulty finding a surgeon who is willing to sterilize them, but poor minority women and welfare mothers are often sterilized against their will. CESA (Committee to End Sterilization Abuse) and other

groups of activists have petitioned the federal and local governments to establish strict guidelines and consent procedures, including a thirty-day waiting period. These guidelines were
adopted, but in many hospitals and clinics they are not being
observed.

Abortion

Men make abortion laws and women have abortions,
whether the law allows them or not. Abortion is a "woman's secret," so statistics on its frequency are not fully reliable.

It is estimated that, worldwide, there are one to two induced
abortions for every four live births. It is thought that in "illegal" countries, such as most of Latin America, abortions are almost as frequent as in legal ones. The notable differences between illegal and legal countries are in the maternal death rate
and the health of women who are sexually active, especially the
poor.

The traditional surgical method is called a "D and C." The
cervical canal is stretched, the contents of the uterus are removed, and the uterus is scraped. An increasingly popular
method, invented in China in the 1950s, involves removal of
the fetus by use of suction created with a pump. Both opera-
tions can be performed under either a local or a general anesthetic, the local (properly administered) being preferred by
most women because it is safer.

Menstrual regulation, a kind of "minisuction" technique, can
be performed without the dilation of the cervical canal but is
not always successful. It must be done in the first two weeks
after a missed period, and it can be painful. Patients who try
this method are advised to have a follow-up pregnancy test two
weeks later.

In early pregnancy, legal abortion does not entail much risk:
the mortality rate in the United States for abortions performed
in the first two months was 0.4 per 100,000 in 1972–73, and it
has declined since. The figures are higher for abortions performed in the second trimester, and a different procedure is

used then—usually the replacement of the amniotic fluid by saline solution to induce labor. The patient will probably suffer some pain, and there are many more chances for complications. An abortion is safest when performed under local anesthesia before the second missed period. Under such circumstances a woman's chances of dying are 1 in 250,000. Where abortion is illegal, the death rate can be as high as 3 per 100.

In the current political climate, and with cutbacks in the availability of legal surgical abortions, it seems imperative for women to eventually have possession of safe home methods that they can manage themselves. In recognition of this, the World Health Organization is collecting information about folk remedies, such as certain herbal teas, that are believed to be effective abortifacients and may be relatively harmless, if certain dose ranges are not exceeded.

The new male attitude

One of the chemists who laid the groundwork for the Pill was asked, many years ago, to help develop a Pill for men.

"Men are too smart to take it," he opined. In fact, most men, most decent men, were unaware until recently of the dangers of the Pill and the IUD. They thought the problems of carefree birth control were settled. A popular gift item of the sixties was a throw pillow that reminded: "Take Your Pill." You don't see them around anymore.

The climate has changed. Informed men worry when the women they love use injurious methods. They want to share responsibility. They are disenchanted with "miracles" and would like to see harmless methods revived and improved.

Luckily, most couples—or individuals—can find a harmless method that is personally acceptable, even aesthetic or pleasure-enhancing. The key is motivation, for as the old song says, "It's what you do with what you got."

CHAPTER 16

Check Out Your Checkup

In most women you don't see a dangerous escalation but we've found that in susceptible women the combination of a little hypertension and a little hyperglycemia, plus a little hyperlipidemia, can be killing.

Dr. William B. Kannel in *Circulation*

We have the medical technology to do it—to eliminate a lot of the high-risk patients—but the argument I get against it is that the less-developed countries don't have the means. They say it would make us look bad abroad to require tests on our women when they can't test theirs.

Dr. William Spellacy

A Pill user's typical checkup is casual—and quick. Her doctor may ask her a few questions about weight gain and menstruation. He may check her breasts, briefly; take her blood pressure; and perform a Pap smear.

But what if she is slowly developing real abnormalities? What if she is on her way toward a blood clot or stroke, a heart attack, diabetes, gallbladder disease, or a fatal disorder of the liver?

Much more elaborate tests could be performed on Pill users, but these tests are somewhat costly. Still, a growing number of scientists argue that the only conscientious way to administer the Pill is in conjunction with these tests. They would not identify all high-risk patients or protect against all Pill-related deaths. According to Dr. Valarie Beral of the London School of Tropical Medicine, the excess mortality of Pill users and former Pill users just from cardiovascular disorders is 39 percent. There are clues to the early onset of such disorders, and perhaps they should be tracked.

Today women who read the patient package inserts know about symptoms to which they should be alert. These include sudden severe headaches; dizziness; double vision; stiffness or paralysis (signs of an impending stroke); redness, pain, or swelling in a limb (signs of a blood clot); chest pain or coughing up blood (signs of a clot in the lung, or pulmonary embolism). Patients know that depression may be associated with the Pill, and that if they become yellow or jaundiced they should stop using it at once. The patient package inserts—which the AMA, pharmaceutical industry, and gynecologists' organizations opposed and fought for almost a decade—are probably helping to save lives. This is the presumption on which the FDA prepared them, and on which the courts sustained the FDA's authority to include them.

But sometimes when the symptoms develop it is already too late. What of the underlying processes that occur before?

Oral contraceptives seem to affect all serum lipids (blood fats), but their effects on triglycerides and very-low-density lipoproteins (LDL) are the most striking and consistent. Younger women are not protected—to the contrary. Dr. William B. Kannel, professor of medicine and chief of the section of preventive medicine and epidemiology at Boston University, notes that the rise in total serum cholesterol and low-density lipoproteins may be particularly notable in young women. In most cases the amount of change is rather modest; in some it is pronounced. But, as Dr. Kannel points out, "We still don't know what the impact of a little shift upward of all these lipids might be in ten or twenty years."

Dr. Kannel suggests that before a woman starts the Pill a "minimum examination" should include finding out whether she has any cardiac problems and determining her blood pressure, blood glucose, and serum cholesterol. If all is clear and the patient starts the medication, the tests should be repeated in six months to a year, to see whether any "alarming changes" are taking place.

To reiterate: *heart problems, blood pressure, blood glucose, and serum cholesterol should all be checked.*

Next there is the question of blood type and clotting factors. In a massive collaborative study performed by scientists in the United States, Sweden, and the United Kingdom, it was found that women with type O blood are less likely to develop clots than those in the A, B, or AB groups. This was true in general, but especially striking where the clots occurred in connection with either Pill use or childbirth. It appears, then, that women with type O blood have less reason to fear Pill-associated clots and, in this regard, are at lower risk from the Pill.

Clotting factors in the blood are extremely complex; the more scientists discover, the less they know. One recent finding is that a normally occurring factor called antithrombin III, which plays an important role in maintaining the fluidity of blood, is adversely affected in 16 percent of women on the Pill. A test that costs about twenty-five dollars, and could be performed at most laboratories, was recently developed by Dr. Stanford Wessler, who was formerly at Harvard and is now at the New York University School of Medicine.

Another caution: before elective surgery and after childbirth, avoid the Pill or any hormone product. Estrogens provoke an eightfold increase in the risk of blood clots associated with surgery or parturition. Stop the Pill for at least a full cycle (some experts advise three months) before elective surgery. After childbirth, do not let your doctor give you estrogens in any form to dry up breast milk. Because of the increased clotting risk, the FDA has withdrawn approval for any use of postpartum estrogen. Apparently many doctors and hospitals either do not know it or do not care, for estrogens are still widely proffered as lactation suppressants. (In truth, they don't even work very well; the non-breast-feeding new mother may be comfortable in the hospital, but once she gets home her breasts are apt to become engorged again. Now, however, it's *her* problem. She will not need to trouble the hospital staff for ice packs, breast pumps, or other palliatives. The best solution, for women who decline to breast-feed, is probably to do just a little bit of nursing and to taper off gradually over the first few weeks. This is healthier for the baby as well as the mother.)

Sometimes a woman on the Pill may need emergency surgery, or may be in an accident. Dr. Wessler and others suggest that, to reduce the risk of clotting, low-dose anticoagulants might be administered.

Finally, if price is no object, women who are determined to take the Pill might have their nutritional profiles taken before starting, three months later, and yearly after that. If they are willing to adjust their diets in accordance with any deficiencies that may arise, they might avert many "nuisance" symptoms as well as some major complications (see Chapter 14). Zinc deficiency may be implicated in stroke, blood clots, skin and reproductive disorders; folic acid deficiency, in anemia and abnormalities of the cervix; vitamin B_6 deficiency, in depression. The Pill, once again, is unlike any other drug in the history of medicine, for it is given to healthy women for long-term use and it subtly alters every body function. Specific dietary steps to help minimize these alterations seem only prudent.

APPENDIX

What follows is the warning that the FDA has ordered to be dispensed with every Pill prescription. If your pharmacist or clinic is not giving it out, tell them that they are breaking the law, and, if you wish, report them to the FDA. The FDA's address is:

Food and Drug Administration
Parklawn Building
5600 Fishers Lane
Rockville, Md. 20857
Commissioner: Jere E. Goyan

The FDA has also mandated that a warning be given to every IUD patient. Whereas it is usually pharmacists who are required to give out the Pill warning, and most of them do comply, it is usually the doctors or clinics who must give out the IUD warning, and a majority—at this writing—are failing to do so. IUD patients who are not offered the warning are also urged to report such noncompliance to the FDA. Copies of such complaints, whether concerning the Pill or the IUD, should also be sent to:

The National Women's Health Network
224 Seventh Street, S.E.
Washington, D.C. 20003
Executive Director: Belita Cowan

The warning you are about to read has been sufficient to make many women draw back from taking the Pill. I have spot-checked with pharmacists who do give out the warning, and they tell me that anywhere from 10 percent to half their customers who walk in with Pill prescriptions are apt, once they've read the warning, to come back and ask if they may return the packet. One pharmacist commented, "I won't even take the money for the Pills until they sit down and read the warning. I don't want to get involved in any lawsuits, and my lawyer advised me that if I don't give the warning out and something happens I could be held to blame. I've put in a chair for my customers to sit and read the Pill warning, and also the warning on Premarin—because even more of those are coming back. They usually say, 'Who needs cancer?' After I put in the chair I had to put a good strong lamp behind it, on account of the print is so small. Sometimes I have to explain the medical terms to my customers. I don't think the FDA tried very hard to get the lay language right."

This warning is a compromise which, as has been noted, was opposed for almost a decade with all the legal and lobbying resources of the pharmaceutical industry, the gynecologists' organizations, and the American Medical Association. Consumer groups were asked to comment on the warning, but most of our suggestions were not observed.

We feel that the weaknesses of the warning include the following:

—It is harder to read than it need be. A glossary of medical terms should be included, and the warning should be available in alternate languages, such as Spanish.

—The special problems of minority groups—for example, the fact that the Pill may be more apt to worsen high blood pressure or sickle-cell anemia in black women—are not noted.

—With methods other than the Pill the worst as well as the best statistics are given. The diaphragm, for example, is listed as having a 2 to 20 percent failure rate. The diaphragm doesn't work if it is left in a bureau drawer, but also the Pill doesn't work if it is left in the medicine cabinet. Nowhere does the warning make clear that the actual failure rate for users of the Pill, even the "combined" high-estrogen Pill, is often much higher than 1 percent and is, in fact, at least 6 percent during the first year. To put it another way, carelessness and human error are taken into account in the figures listed here for the barrier methods but are ignored in the figures given for the Pill. Instead, the "ideal" statistics are reiterated.

Mention of the common drugs that interact with the Pill and make it less effective is also omitted. Nor is it frankly stated that the diaphragm, properly fitted and conscientiously used, can be *just as reliable* as the Pill.

—The FDA also makes the curious assumption that "except for the IUD, effective use of [other] methods requires somewhat more effort than simply taking a single pill every day. . . ."

A great many women *do not* have sex relations on a regular basis. A woman may, for example, have a lover or husband from whom she is geographically separated. For such women, taking the Pill every day—even leaving aside the question of risk—may take a lot more "effort" than using a barrier method from time to time.

—Death rates are given for cardiovascular and other disorders, but not hospitalization rates. As many as one in five hundred Pill users winds up in the hospital every year for treatment of some serious complication. Very often there are permanent effects.

—The warning does not disclose that death rates remain substantially higher among former users of the Pill than among comparable women who never took it. Some of the changes it brings appear to stay with women for life, even if they escape immediate disturbances.

—The so-called nuisance side effects are not discussed at sufficient length. It is not mentioned, for example, that many vaginal, bladder, and herpes infections do not seem to clear up unless a woman stops using the Pill.

—The warning hedges on the seriousness of cancer risks. It does not, for example, mention the manifold increase in early cervical cancers that is now well established to exist in women who take the Pill.

—The metabolic and nutritional disturbances are minimized. These were mentioned in some versions of the warning and then, for unexplained reasons, taken out. Consider the situation with folic acid. Deaths from folic-acid-deficiency anemia have been reported in Pill users with some frequency. The negative effects of folic-acid deficiency on the reproductive organs of Pill users have also become increasingly clear. In March 1980 the Center for Population Research's *Progress Report* stated:

> Preliminary results from a clinical trial of dietary folate [an essential nutrient] supplementation in women using oral contraceptives suggests that folate supplementation prevents progression of cervical dysplasia [abnormalities] to carcinoma, and may effect regression.

Government-financed scientists are working on the possibility that increased folic acid in the diet may actually prevent certain cancers in users of the Pill. Yet the FDA doesn't warn women that either these cancers or the folic acid deficiencies even exist!

—The warning tells women who miss a period to go on taking

their pills. Many critics feel that this is awful advice and that a pregnancy test should be performed immediately. If the woman is pregnant and wants an abortion, the abortion will be later and more dangerous if she follows the FDA's advice. If she wants to have the baby, her child is exposed to further hormones that may cause birth defects.

—The warning hedges on whether DES daughters should take the Pill. Many DES researchers think that the Pill would be highly inadvisable for any young woman exposed to DES in the womb. Hormones are being added to more hormones, which have already damaged her enough.

With all these reservations, we think that the warning is a great advance toward the rights, and autonomy, of female patients. We hope that all prescription drugs will soon be marketed with comprehensive patient labeling. More people are hospitalized each year in the United States from side effects of drugs prescribed by their doctors than from side effects of "street" or illicit drugs.

DETAILED PATIENT LABELING FOR ORAL CONTRACEPTIVES REQUIRED BY THE FOOD AND DRUG ADMINISTRATION

What you should know about oral contraceptives

Oral contraceptives ("the Pill") are the most effective way (except for sterilization) to prevent pregnancy. They are also convenient and, for most women, free of serious or unpleasant side effects. Oral contraceptives must always be taken under the continuous supervision of a physician.

It is important that any woman who considers using an oral contraceptive understand the risks involved. Although the oral contraceptives have important advantages over other methods of contraception, they have certain risks that no other method has. Only you can decide whether the advantages are worth these risks. This leaflet will tell you about the most important risks. It will explain how you can help your doctor prescribe the Pill as safely as possible by telling him about yourself and being alert for the earliest signs of trouble. And it will tell you how to use the Pill properly, so that it will be as effective as possible. There is more detailed information available in the leaflet prepared for doctors. Your pharmacist can show you a copy; you may need your doctor's help in understanding parts of it.

Who should not use oral contraceptives

A. If you have any of the following conditions, you should not use the Pill:

1. Clots in the legs or lungs.
2. Angina pectoris.
3. Known or suspected cancer of the breast or sex organs.
4. Unusual vaginal bleeding that has not yet been diagnosed.
5. Known or suspected pregnancy.

B. If you have had any of the following conditions, you should not use the Pill:

1. Heart attack or stroke.
2. Clots in the legs or lungs.

C. Cigarette smoking increases the risk of serious adverse effects on the heart and blood vessels from oral-contraceptive use. This risk increases with age and with heavy smoking (15 or more cigarettes per day) and is quite marked in women over 35 years of age. Women who use oral contraceptives should not smoke.

D. If you have scanty or irregular periods or are a young woman without a regular cycle, you should use another method of contraception because, if you use the Pill, you may have difficulty becoming pregnant or may fail to have menstrual periods after discontinuing the Pill.

Deciding to use oral contraceptives

If you do not have any of the conditions listed above and are thinking about using oral contraceptives, to help you decide, you need information about the advantages and risks of oral contraceptives and of other contraceptive methods as well. This leaflet describes the advantages and risks of oral contraceptives. Except for sterilization, the IUD, and abortion, which have their own exclusive risks, the only risks of other methods of contraception are those due to pregnancy should the method fail. Your doctor can answer questions you may have with respect to other methods of contraception. He can also answer any questions you may have after reading this leaflet on oral contraceptives.

1. What Oral Contraceptives Are and How They Work. Oral contraceptives are of two types. The most common, often simply called "the Pill," is a combination of an estrogen and a progestogen, the two kinds of female hormones. The amount of estrogen and progestogen can vary, but the amount of estrogen is most important because both the effectiveness and some of the dangers of oral contraceptives are related to the amount of estrogen. This kind of oral contraceptive works principally by preventing release of an egg from the ovary. When the amount of estrogen is 50 micrograms or more, and the Pill is taken as directed, oral contraceptives are more than 99% effective (i.e., there would be less than 1 pregnancy if 100 women used the Pill for 1 year). Pills that contain 20 to 35 micrograms of estrogen vary slightly in effectiveness, ranging from 98% to more than 99% effective.

The second type of oral contraceptive, often called the "minipill," contains only a progestogen. It works in part by preventing release of an egg from the ovary but also by keeping sperm from reaching the egg and by making the uterus (womb) less receptive to any fertilized egg that reaches it. The minipill is less effective than the combination oral contraceptive, about 97% effective. In addition, the progestogen-only pill has a tendency to cause irregular bleeding which may be quite inconvenient, or cessation of bleeding entirely. The progestogen-only pill is used despite its lower effectiveness in the hope that it will prove not to have some of the serious side effects of the estrogen-containing pill (see below), but it is not yet certain that the minipill does in fact have fewer serious side effects. The discussion below, while based mainly on information about the combination pills, should be considered to apply as well to the minipill.

2. Other Nonsurgical Ways to Prevent Pregnancy. As this leaflet will explain, oral contraceptives have several serious risks. Other methods of contraception have lesser risks or none at all. They are also less effective than oral contraceptives, but, used properly, may be effective enough for many women.

The following table gives reported pregnancy rates (the number of women out of 100 who would become pregnant in 1 year) for these methods:

Pregnancies per 100 women per year

Intrauterine device (IUD), less than 1–6; Diaphragm with spermicidal products (creams or jellies), 2–20; Condom (rubber), 3–36; Aerosol foams, 2–29; Jellies and creams, 4–36; Periodic abstinence (rhythm) all types, less than 1–47:

1. Calendar method, 14–47;
2. Temperature method, 1–20;
3. Temperature method—intercourse only in post-ovulatory phase, less than 1–7;
4. Mucus method, 1–25;

No contraception, 60–80.

The figures (except for the IUD) vary widely because people differ in how well they use each method. Very faithful users of the various methods obtain very good results, except for users of the calendar method of periodic abstinence (rhythm). Except for the IUD, effective use of these methods requires somewhat more effort than simply taking a single pill every day, but it is an effort that many couples undertake successfully. Your doctor can tell you a great deal more about these methods of contraception.

3. The Dangers of Oral Contraceptives.

a. *Circulatory disorders (abnormal blood clotting and stroke due to hemorrhage).* Blood clots (in various blood vessels of the body) are the most common of the serious side effects of oral contraceptives. A clot can result in a stroke (if the clot is in the brain), a heart attack (if the clot is in a blood vessel of the heart), or a pulmonary embolus (a clot which forms in the legs or pelvis, then breaks off and travels to the lungs). Any of these can be fatal. Clots also occur rarely in the blood vessels of the eye, resulting in blindness or impairment of vision in that eye. There is evidence that the risk of clotting increases with higher estrogen doses. It is therefore important to keep the dose of estrogen as low as possible, so long as the oral contraceptive used has an acceptable pregnancy rate and doesn't cause unacceptable changes in the menstrual pattern. Furthermore, cigarette smoking by oral-contraceptive users increases the risk of serious adverse effects on the heart and blood vessels. This risk increases with age and with heavy smoking (15 or more cigarettes per day) and begins to become quite marked in women over 35 years of age. For this reason, women who use oral contraceptives should not smoke. The risk of abnormal clotting increases with age in both users and nonusers of oral contraceptives, but the increased risk from the contraceptive appears to be present at all ages. For oral-contraceptive users in general, it has been estimated that in women between the ages of 15 and 34 the risk of death due to a circulatory disorder is about 1 in 12,000 per year, whereas for nonusers the rate is about 1 in 50,000 per year. In the age group 35 to 44, the risk is estimated to be about 1 in 2,500 per year for oral-contraceptive users and about 1 in 10,000 per year for nonusers.

Even without the Pill the risk of having a heart attack increases with age and is also increased by such heart attack risk factors as high blood pressure, high cholesterol, obesity, diabetes, and cigarette smoking. Without any risk factors present, the use of oral contraceptives alone may double the risk of heart attack. However, the combination of cigarette smoking, especially heavy smoking, and oral-contraceptive use greatly increases the risk of heart attack. Oral-contraceptive users who smoke are about 5 times more likely to have a heart attack than users who do not smoke and about 10 times more likely to have a heart attack than nonusers who do not smoke. It has been estimated that users between the ages of 30 and 39 who smoke have about a 1 in 10,000 chance each year of having a fatal heart attack compared to about a 1 in 50,000 chance in users who do not smoke, and about a 1 in 100,000 chance in nonusers who do not smoke. In the age group 40 to 44, the risk is about 1 in 1,700 per year for users who smoke compared to about 1 in 10,000 for users who do not smoke and to about 1 in 14,000 per year for nonusers who do not smoke. Heavy smoking (about 15 cigarettes or more a day) further increases the risk. If you do not smoke and have none of the other heart attack risk factors described above, you will have a smaller risk than listed. If you have several heart attack risk factors, the risk may be considerably greater than listed. In addition to blood-clotting disorders, it has been estimated that women taking oral contraceptives are twice as likely as nonusers to have a stroke due to rupture of a blood vessel in the brain.

b. *Formation of tumors.* Studies have found that when certain animals are given the female sex hormone, estrogen, which is an ingredient of oral contraceptives, continuously for long periods, cancers may develop in the breast, cervix, vagina, and liver. These findings suggest that oral contraceptives may cause cancer in humans. However, studies to date in women taking currently marketed oral contraceptives have not confirmed that oral contraceptives cause cancer in humans. Several studies have found no increase in breast cancer in users, although one study suggested oral contraceptives might cause an increase in breast cancer in women who already have benign breast disease (e.g., cysts).

Women with a strong family history of breast cancer or who have breast nodules, fibrocystic disease, or abnormal mammograms or who were exposed to DES (diethylstilbestrol), an estrogen, during their mother's pregnancy must be followed very closely by their doctors if they choose to use oral contraceptives instead of another method of contraception. Many studies have shown that women taking oral contraceptives have less risk of getting benign breast disease than those who have not used oral contraceptives. Recently, strong evidence has emerged that estrogens (one component of oral contraceptives), when given for periods of more than one year to women after the menopause, increase the risk of cancer of the uterus (womb). There is also some evidence that a kind of oral contraceptive which is no longer marketed, the sequential oral contraceptive, may increase the risk of cancer of the uterus. There remains no evidence, however, that the oral contraceptives now available increase the risk of this cancer. Oral contraceptives do cause, although rarely, a benign (nonmalignant) tumor of the liver. These tumors do not spread, but they may rupture and cause internal bleeding, which may be fatal. A few cases of cancer of the liver have been reported in women using oral contraceptives, but it is not yet known whether the drug caused them.

c. *Dangers to a developing child if oral contraceptives are used in or immediately preceding pregnancy.* Oral contraceptives should not be taken by pregnant women because they may damage the developing child. An increased risk of birth defects, including heart defects and limb defects, has been associated with the use of sex hormones, including oral contraceptives, in pregnancy. In addition, the developing female child whose mother has received DES (diethylstilbestrol), an estrogen, during pregnancy has a risk of getting cancer of the vagina or cervix in her teens or young adulthood. This risk is estimated to be about 1 in 1,000 exposures or less. Abnormalities of the urinary and sex organs have been reported in male offspring so exposed. It is possible that other estrogens, such as the estrogens in oral contraceptives, could have the same effect in the child if the mother takes them during pregnancy.

If you stop taking oral contraceptives to become pregnant, your doctor may recommend that you use another method of contraception for a short while. The reason for this is that there is evidence from studies in women who have had "miscarriages" soon after stopping the Pill, that the lost fetuses are more likely to be abnormal. Whether there is an overall increase in "miscarriage" in women who become pregnant soon after stopping the Pill as compared with women who do not use the Pill is not known, but it is possible that there may be. If, however, you do become pregnant soon after stopping oral contraceptives, and do not have a miscarriage, there is no evidence that the baby has an increased risk of being abnormal.

d. *Gallbladder disease.* Women who use oral contraceptives have a greater risk than nonusers of having gallbladder disease requiring surgery. The increased risk may first appear within 1 year of use and may double after 4 or 5 years of use.

e. *Other side effects of oral contraceptives.* Some women using oral contraceptives experience unpleasant side effects that are not dangerous and are not likely to damage their health. Some of these may be temporary. Your breasts may feel tender, nausea and vomiting may occur, you may gain or lose weight, and your ankles may swell. A spotty darkening of the skin, particularly of the face, is possible and may persist. You may notice unexpected vaginal bleeding or changes in your menstrual period. Irregular bleeding is frequently seen when using the minipill or combination oral contraceptives containing less than 50 micrograms of estrogen.

More serious side effects include worsening of migraine, asthma, epilepsy, and kidney or heart disease because of a tendency for water to be retained in the body when oral contraceptives are used.

Other side effects are growth of preexisting fibroid tumors of the uterus; mental depression; and liver problems with jaundice (yellowing of the skin). Your doctor may find that levels of sugar and fatty substances in your blood are elevated; the long-term effects of these changes are not known. Some women develop high blood pressure while taking oral contraceptives, which ordinarily returns to the original levels when the oral contraceptive is stopped. Other reactions, although not proved to be caused by oral contraceptives, are occasionally reported. These include more frequent urination and some discomfort when urinating, nervousness, dizziness, some loss of scalp hair, an increase in body hair, an increase or decrease in sex drive, appetite changes, cataracts, and a need for a change in contact lens prescription, or inability to use contact lenses.

After you stop using oral contraceptives, there may be a delay before you are able to become pregnant or before you resume having menstrual periods. This is especially true of women who had irregular menstrual cycles prior to the use of oral contraceptives. As discussed previously, your doctor may recommend that you wait a short while after stopping the Pill before you try to become pregnant. During this time, use another form of contraception. You should consult your physician before resuming use of oral contraceptives after childbirth, especially if you plan to nurse your baby. Drugs in oral contraceptives are known to appear in the milk, and the long-range effect on infants is not known at this time. Furthermore, oral contraceptives may cause a decrease in your milk supply as well as in the quality of the milk.

4. Comparison of the Risks of Oral Contraceptives and Other Contraceptive Methods. The many studies on the risks and effectiveness of oral contraceptives and other methods of contraception have been analyzed to estimate the risk of death associated with various methods of contraception. This risk has two parts: (a) the risk of the method itself (e.g., the risk that oral contraceptives will cause death due to abnormal clotting), and (b) the risk of death due to pregnancy or abortion in the event the method fails. The results of this analysis are shown in the bar graph. The height of the bars is the number of deaths per 100,000 women each year. There are six sets of bars, each set referring to a specific age group of women. Within each set of bars, there is a single bar for each of the different contraceptive methods. For oral contraceptives, there are two bars—one for smokers and the other for nonsmokers. The analysis is based on present knowledge, and new information could, of course, alter it. The analysis shows that the risk of death from all methods of birth control is low and below that associated with childbirth, except for oral contraceptives in women over 40 who smoke. It shows that the lowest risk of death is associated with the condom or diaphragm (traditional contraception) backed up by early abortion in case of failure of the condom or diaphragm to pre-

vent pregnancy. Also, at any age the risk of death (due to unexpected pregnancy) from the use of traditional contraception, even without a backup of abortion, is generally the same as or less than that from use of oral contraceptives.

How to use oral contraceptives as safely and effectively as possible, once you have decided to use them

1. What to Tell Your Doctor.
You can make use of the Pill as safely as possible by telling your doctor if you have any of the following:
a. Conditions that mean you should not use oral contraceptives:
Clots in the legs or lungs.
Clots in the legs or lungs in the past.
A stroke, heart attack, or angina pectoris.
Known or suspected cancer of the breast or sex organs.
Unusual vaginal bleeding that has not yet been diagnosed.
Known or suspected pregnancy.
b. Conditions that your doctor will want to watch closely or which might cause him to suggest another method of contraception:
A family history of breast cancer.
Breast nodules, fibrocystic disease of the breast, or an abnormal mammogram.
Diabetes.
High blood pressure.
High cholesterol.
Cigarette smoking.
Migraine headaches.
Heart or kidney disease.
Epilepsy.
Mental depression.
Fibroid tumors of the uterus.
Gallbladder disease.
c. Once you are using oral contraceptives, you should be alert for signs of a serious adverse effect and call your doctor if they occur:
Sharp pain in the chest, coughing blood, or sudden shortness of breath (indicating possible clots in the lungs).
Pain in the calf (possible clot in the leg).
Crushing chest pain or heaviness (indicating possible heart attack).

Sudden severe headache or vomiting, dizziness or fainting, disturbance of vision or speech, or weakness or numbness in an arm or leg (indicating a possible stroke).

Sudden partial or complete loss of vision (indicating a possible clot in the eye).

Breast lumps (you should ask your doctor to show you how to examine your own breasts).

Severe pain in the abdomen (indicating a possible ruptured tumor of the liver).

Severe depression.

Yellowing of the skin (jaundice).

2. How to Take the Pill So That It Is Most Effective.

To achieve maximum contraceptive effectiveness, oral contraceptives must be taken exactly as directed and at intervals not exceeding 24 hours. It is recommended that tablets be taken at the same time each day, preferably after the evening meal or at bedtime. Taking them on a definite schedule will decrease the chance of forgetting a tablet and also help keep the proper amount of medication in your system.

At times there may be no menstrual period after a cycle of pills. Therefore, if you miss one menstrual period but have taken the pills *exactly as you were supposed to*, continue as usual into the next cycle. If you have not taken the pills correctly and miss a menstrual period, or if you are taking minipills and it is 45 days or more from the start of your last menstrual period you may be pregnant and should stop taking oral contraceptives until your doctor determines whether or not you are pregnant. Until you can get to your doctor, use another form of contraception. If two consecutive menstrual periods are missed, you should stop taking pills until it is determined whether you are pregnant. If you do become pregnant while using oral contraceptives, you should discuss the risks to the developing child with your doctor.

3. Periodic Examination.

Your doctor will take a complete medical and family history before prescribing oral contraceptives. At that time and about once a year thereafter, he will generally examine your blood pressure, breasts, abdomen, and pelvic organs (including a Papanicolaou smear, i.e., test for cancer).

Summary

Oral contraceptives are the most effective method, except sterilization, for preventing pregnancy. Other methods, when used conscientiously, are also very effective and have fewer risks. The serious risks of oral contraceptives are uncommon, and the "Pill" is a very convenient method of preventing pregnancy. If you have certain conditions or have had these conditions in the past, you should not use oral contraceptives, because the risk is too great. These conditions are listed in the leaflet. If you do not have these conditions, and decide to use the "Pill," please read the leaflet carefully so that you can use the "Pill" most safely and effectively.

Based on his or her assessment of your medical needs, your doctor has prescribed this drug for you. Do not give the drug to anyone else.

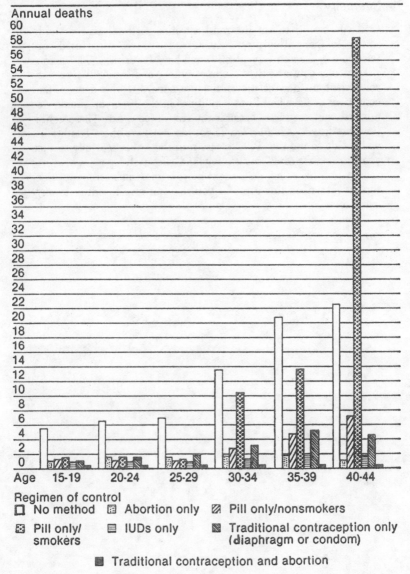

Figure 1. Estimated annual number of deaths associated with control of fertility and no control per 100,000 nonsterile women, by regimen of control and age of woman.

Notes and References

CHAPTER 1   WHO TAKES THE PILL?

SIDE EFFECTS:

Joint hearings before the Subcommittee on Health of the Committee on Labor and Public Welfare and the Subcommittee on Administrative Practice and Procedure of the Committee on the Judiciary, U. S. Senate, 94th Congress, 1975 (Kennedy hearings).

Hearings before the Subcommittee on Monopoly of the Select Committee on Small Business, U. S. Senate, 91st Congress, 1970 (Nelson hearings).

Royal College of General Practitioners, *Oral Contraception and Health: An Interim Report* (New York: Pitman, 1974).

H. A. Salhanick, D. M. Kipnis, and R. L. Vande Wiele, eds., *Metabolic Effects of Gonadal Hormones and Contraceptive Steroids* (New York: Plenum, 1969).

M. P. Vessey, K. McPherson, and B. Johnson, "Mortality among women participating in the Oxford/Family Planning Association contraceptive study," *Lancet* 2(8041): 731–33 (Oct. 8, 1977).

V. Wynn, "Vitamins and contraceptive use," *Lancet* 1:561 (1975).

DEATH RATES:

Department of Health, Education, and Welfare, *Facts of Life and Death* (Nov. 1978).

STERILIZATION AND PRESCRIPTIONS IN CLINICS:

Population Reports, Ser. A, No. 5 (Jan. 1979), p. 136.

CANCER RISK:

R. J. Ryan, "Cancer risk and estrogen use in menopause," *New England Journal of Medicine* 293:1164–67 (1975).

D. C. Smith et al., "Association of exogenous estrogens and endometrial carcinoma," *New England Journal of Medicine* 293:1200–1 (1975).

N. S. Weiss, "Risks and benefits of estrogen use," *New England Journal of Medicine* 293:1164–67 (1975).

Food and Drug Administration, *Drug Bulletin* (Feb./Mar. 1976).

TEENAGERS:

M. Zelnick, Y. J. Kim, and J. F. Kantner, "Probabilities of intercourse and conception among U.S. teenage women, 1971 and 1976," *Family Planning Perspectives* 3X 2:3 (May/June 1979).

INFERTILITY:

M. Vessey, R. Doll, et al., "A long-term follow-up study of women using different methods of contraception: an interim report," *Journal of Biosocial Science* 8(4):375–427 (Oct. 1976).

CHAPTER 3   BLOOD-CLOTTING: NUMBER ONE DANGER

Food and Drug Administration, patient package insert, oral contraceptives; see Appendix for text.

D. H. Lawson, J. F. Davidson, and H. Jick, "Oral contraceptive use and venous thromboembolism: absence of an effect of smoking," *British Medical Journal* 2:729–30 (1977).

H. Jick, J. Porter, and K. J. Rothman, "Oral contraceptives and nonfatal stroke in healthy young women," *Annals of Internal Medicine* 89:58–60 (July 1978).

Collaborative Group for the Study of Stroke in Young Women, "Oral contraceptives and stroke in young women," *Journal of the American Medical Association* 231:718–22 (1975).

M. C. Cole, "Strokes in young women using oral contraceptives," *Archives of Internal Medicine* 120:551–55 (1967).

Center for Population Research, National Institutes of Health (HEW and Public Health Service), *The Walnut Creek Contraceptive Drug Study* 1:201 (1974).

Royal College of General Practitioners, *Oral Contraception and Health* (1974), p. 48.

T. N. A. Jeffcoate et al., "Management of normal pregnancy, labor and puerperium: puerperal thromboembolism in relation to the inhibition of lactation by oestrogen therapy," *British Medical Journal* 4:222 (1968).

W. H. W. Inman, M. P. Vessey, et al., "Thromboembolic disease and the steroidal content of oral contraceptives: A report to the Committee on the Safety of Drugs," *British Medical Journal* 2:203–9 (1970).

P. D. Stolley et al., "Thrombosis with low-estrogen oral contraceptives," *American Journal of Epidemiology* 102:197–208 (1975).

P. E. Sartwell et al., "Thromboembolism and oral contraceptives," *American Journal of Epidemiology* 90:365–80 (1969).

Nelson hearings, 1970, I:6135–56.

Population Reports, Ser. A, No. 5 (Jan. 1979), pp. 133–86.

N. Aikjaersig, A. Fletcher, and R. Burstein, "Association between oral contraceptive use and thromboembolism: a new approach to its investigation based on plasma fibrinogen chromatography," *American Journal of Obstetrics and Gynecology* 122(2):199–211 (May 15, 1975).

S. Sager, J. D. Stamatakis, D. P. Thomas, and V. V. Kakkar, "Oral contraceptives, antithrombin III activity and deep-vein thrombosis," *Lancet* 1(7958):509–11 (Mar. 6, 1976).

CHAPTER 4   HEART DISEASE AND THE PILL

J. I. Mann and W. H. W. Inman, "Oral contraceptives and death from myocardial infarction," *British Medical Journal* 2(5965):245–48 (May 3, 1975).

J. I. Mann, W. H. W. Inman, and M. Thorogood, "Oral contraceptive use in older women and fatal myocardial infarction," *British Medical Journal* 2(8033):445–47 (Aug. 21, 1976).

J. I. Mann, M. Thorogood, W. E. Waters, and C. Powell, "Oral contraceptives and myocardial infarction in young women: a further report," *British Medical Journal* 2(5984):631–32 (Sept. 13, 1975).

J. I. Mann, M. P. Vessey, M. Thorogood, and R. Doll, "Myocardial infarction in young women with special reference to oral contraceptive practice," *British Medical Journal* 2(5965):241–45 (May 3, 1975).

A. C. Arntzenius, C. M. vanGent, H. van der Voort, C. I. Stegerhoek, and K. Styblo, "Reduced high-density lipoprotein in women aged 40–41 using oral contraceptives," *Lancet* 1(8076):1222–23 (June 10, 1978).

D. D. Bradley, J. Wingerd, D. B. Petit, R. M. Krauss, and S. Ramcharan, "Serum high-density lipoprotein cholesterol in women using oral contraceptives, estrogen and progestins," *New England Journal of Medicine* 299(1):17–20 (July 6, 1978).

T. Gordon, W. P. Castelli, M. C. Hjortland, W. B. Kannel, and T. R. Dawber, "High-density lipoproteins as a protective factor against coronary heart disease: the Framingham study," *American Journal of Medicine* 62:707–14 (1977).

Inman, Vessey, et al., "Thromboembolic disease . . ." (1970).

R. M. Krauss, F. T. Lingren, A. Silvers, R. Jutagir, and D. D. Bradley, "Changes in high-density lipoproteins in women on oral contraceptive drugs," *Clinica Chimica Acta* 80(3):465–70 (Nov. 1, 1977).

J. D. Shelton and D. Petitti, "Formulation-dependent effect of oral contraceptives on HDL-cholesterol" (letter to the editor), *Lancet* 2(8091) (Sept. 23, 1978).

Population Reports, Ser. A, No. 5 (Jan. 1979), p. 150.

Center for Population Research, *The Walnut Creek . . . Study* (1974).

Royal College of General Practitioners, *Oral Contraception and Health* (1974).

J. R. Fisch and J. Frank, "Oral contraceptives and blood pressure," *Journal of the American Medical Association* 237(23):2499–503 (June 6, 1977).

J. A. Pritchard and S. A. Pritchard, "Blood pressure response to estrogen-progestin oral contraceptives after pregnancy-induced hypertension," *American Journal of Obstetrics and Gynecology* 129(7):733–39 (Dec. 1, 1977).

R. Hoover, C. Bain, P. Cole, and B. MacMahon, "Oral contraceptive use: association with frequency of hospitalization and chronic disease risk indicators," *American Journal of Public Health* 68(4):335–41 (April 1978).

H. W. Ory, "Association between oral contraceptives and myocardial infarction: a review," *Journal of the American Medical Association* 237(24):2619–22 (June 13, 1977).

A. K. Jain, "Mortality risk association with the use of oral contraceptives," *Studies in Family Planning* 8(3):50–54 (Mar. 1977).

C. Tietze, "New estimates of mortality association with fertility control," *Family Planning Perspectives* 9(2):74–75 (Mar./Apr. 1977).

M. P. Vessey, K. McPherson, and B. Johnson, "Mortality among women participating in the Oxford/Family Planning Association contraceptive study," *Lancet* 2(8047):731–33 (Oct. 8, 1977).

H. Frederiksen and R. T. Ravenholt, "Oral contraceptives and thromboembolic disease" (letter to the editor), *British Medical Journal* 4(5633):770 (Dec. 21, 1968).

H. Frederiksen and R. T. Ravenholt, "Thromboembolism, oral contraceptives and cigarettes," *Public Health Reports* 85(3):197–205 (Mar. 1970).

Population Reports, Ser. L, No. 1 (Mar. 1979).

Royal College of General Practitioners' Oral Contraception Study, "Mortality among oral contraceptive users," *Lancet* 2(8041):727–31 (Oct. 8, 1977).

W. H. W. Inman and M. P. Vessey, "Investigation of deaths from pulmonary, coronary and cerebral thrombosis and embolism in women of childbearing age," *British Medical Journal* 2(5599):193–99 (Apr. 27, 1968).

CHAPTER 5   STROKES AND THE PILL

U. S. Bureau of the Census, *Statistical Abstract of the United States*, 99th Edition (Washington, D.C.: U. S. Government Printing Office, 1978).

U. S. National Center for Health Statistics, Department of Health, Education, and Welfare, *Facts of Life and Death* (Nov. 1978).

Royal College of General Practitioners, *Oral Contraception and Health* (1974).

Royal College of General Practitioners, "Mortality among oral contraceptive users" (1977).

Royal College of General Practitioners' Oral Contraception Study, "Oral contraceptives, venous thrombosis, and varicose veins," *Journal of the Royal College of General Practitioners* 28(192):393–99 (July 1978).

Center for Population Research, *The Walnut Creek . . . Study* (1974). See also notes from Chapters 3 and 4, as well as:

V. Beral, "Cardiovascular disease mortality trends and oral contraceptive use in young women," *Lancet* 2:1047–51 (1976).

W. H. W. Inman and M. P. Vessey, "Investigation of deaths from pulmonary, coronary and cerebral thrombosis and embolism in women of childbearing age," *British Medical Journal* 2(5599):193–99 (Apr. 1968).

V. A. Drill and D. W. Calhoun, "Oral contraceptives and thromboembolic disease," *Journal of the American Medical Association* 206:77–84 (1968).

CHAPTER 6   CANCER AND THE PILL

W. U. Gardner, "Estrogens in carcinogenesis," *Archives of Pathology* 27:139–70 (1939).

L. Loeb, "Significance of hormones in the origin of cancer," *Journal of the U.S. National Cancer Institute* 1:169–95 (1940).

R. Hertz, "The role of steroid hormones in the etiology and pathogenesis of cancer," *American Journal of Obstetrics and Gynecology* 98:1013–19 (1967).

E. Fasal and R. S. Paffenbarger, "Oral contraceptives as related to cancer and benign lesions of the breast," *Journal of the National Cancer Institute* 55:4 (1975).

E. Stern, A. B. Forsythe, and C. F. Coffelt, "Steroid contraceptive use and cervical dysplasia: increased risk of progression," *Science* 196(4297) (June 24, 1977).

Population Reports, Ser. A, No. 4 (May 1977), pp. 69–90.

Armed Forces Institute of Pathology, Hepatic Branch and Center for Disease Control, Bureau of Epidemiology, Family Planning Evaluation Division, "Increased risk of hepatocellular adenoma in women with long-term use of oral contraceptives," *Morbidity and Mortality Weekly Report* 26(36):293–94 (Sept. 9, 1977).

W. L. Ramseur and M. R. Cooper, "Asymptomatic liver cell adenomas: another case of resolution after discontinuance of oral contraceptive use," *Journal of the American Medical Association* 239(16):1647–48 (Apr. 21, 1978).

H. A. Edmondson, T. B. Reynolds, B. Henderson, and B. Benton, "Regression of liver cell adenomas associated with oral contraceptives," *Annals of Internal Medicine* 86(2):180–82 (Feb. 1977).

Center for Population Research, *The Walnut Creek . . . Study* (1974).

Population Reports, Ser. A, No. 5 (Jan. 1979).

R. S. Paffenbarger, *Cancer* 39:1887 (1979).

M. Vessey and R. Doll, *British Medical Journal* 1:1755 (1979).

R. Hoover, personal communication (Apr. 1980).

Population Reports, Ser. A, No. 2 (Mar. 1975).

R. S. Paffenbarger, E. Fasal, M. E. Simmons, and J. B. Kampert, "Cancer risk as related to oral contraceptives during fertile years," *Cancer* 39(4, Suppl.):1887–91 (1977).

V. A. LiVolsi, B. V. Stadel, J. L. Kelsey, T. R. Holford, and C. White, "Fibrocystic breast disease in oral contraceptive users: a histopathological evaluation of epithelial atypia," *New England Journal of Medicine* 299(8):381–85 (Aug. 24, 1978).

M. R. Melamed et al., "Prevalence rates of uterine cervical carcinoma in situ for women using the diaphragm or oral contraceptives," *British Medical Journal* 3:195 (1969).

M. Vessey, R. Doll, R. Peto, B. Johnson, and P. Wiggins, "A long-term follow-up study of women using different methods of contraception: an interim report," *Journal of Biosocial Science* 8(4):375–427 (Oct. 1976).

G. G. Wied et al., "Statistical evaluation of the effect of hormonal contraceptives on the cytologic smear pattern," *Obstetrics and Gynecology* 27:327 (1966).

H. B. Taylor, N. S. Irey, and H. J. Morris, "Atypical endocervical hyperplasia in women taking oral contraceptives," *Journal of the American Medical Association* 202:637 (1967).

S. H. Geist et al., "Are estrogens carcinogenic in the human female?," *American Journal of Obstetrics and Gynecology* 41:29–36 (1941).

M. Candy and M. R. Abel, "Progestogen-induced adenomatous hyperplasia of the uterine cervix," *Journal of the American Medical Association* 202:323 (1968).

S. A. Gall, C. H. Bourgeois, and R. McGuire, "The morphologic effects of oral contraceptive agents on the cervix," *Journal of the American Medical Association* 207:2243–47 (1969).

CHAPTER 7   DIABETES AND THE PILL

V. Wynn and J. W. H. Doar, "Longitudinal studies of the effects of oral contraceptive therapy on plasma glucose, non-esterified fatty acid, insulin and blood pyruvate levels during oral and intravenous glucose tolerance tests," in *Metabolic Effects of Gonadal Hormones and Contraceptive Steroids*, H. A. Salhanick, D. M. Kipnis, and R. L. Vande Wiele, eds. (New York: Plenum, 1969), pp. 157–77.

P. Beck, "Effects of gonadal hormones and contraceptive steroids on glucose and insulin metabolism," in *Metabolic Effects*, Salhanick et al., eds. (1969).

W. N. Spellacy, "The effects of ovarian steroids on glucose, insulin and growth hormone," in *Metabolic Effects*, Salhanick et al., eds. (1969).

H. Gershberg, H. Hulse, and Z. Javier, "Hypertriglyceridemia during treatment with estrogen and oral contraceptives," *Obstetrics and Gynecology* 31:188–91 (1968).

Editorial, *Lancet* 2:783–84 (1969).

W. N. Spellacy, "A review of carbohydrate metabolism and the oral contraceptives," *American Journal of Obstetrics and Gynecology* 104:448–60 (1969).

W. N. Spellacy, "Progesten and estrogen effects on carbohydrate metabolism," in *Uterine Contraction: Side Effects of Steroidal Contraception*, J. B. Josimovich, ed. (New York: Wiley, 1973), pp. 327–41.

W. N. Spellacy, "Metabolic effects of oral contraceptives," *Clinical Obstetrics and Gynecology* 17:53–64 (1974).

V. Wynn and J. W. H. Doar, "Some effects of oral contraceptives on carbohydrate metabolism," *Lancet* 2:715 (1966).

V. Wynn, J. W. H. Doar, and G. L. Mills, "Some effects of oral contraceptives on serum lipid and lipoprotein levels," *Lancet* 2:720 (1966).

V. Wynn, "Some metabolic effects of oral contraceptives," *Clinical Trials Journal* 5:171 (1968).

J. W. H. Doar, V. Wynn, and D. G. Cramp, "Blood pyruvate and plasma glucose levels during oral and intravenous glucose tolerance tests in obese and non-obese women," *Metabolism* 7:690 (1968).

V. Wynn, G. L. Mills, J. W. H. Doar, and T. Stokes, "Fasting serum triglyceride, cholesterol and lipoprotein levels during oral contraceptive therapy," *Lancet* 2:756–60 (1969).

W. N. Spellacy, "Carbohydrate metabolism in male infertility and female fertility-control patients," *Fertility and Sterility* 27:1132–39 (1976).

Dr. William Spellacy, personal communication (Nov. 1979).

W. N. Spellacy, R. E. Newton, and S. A. Berk, "The effects of a 'low-estrogen' oral contraceptive on carbohydrate metabolism during six months of treatment: a preliminary report of blood glucose and plasma insulin values," *Fertility and Sterility* 28:885–87 (1977).

Population Reports, Ser. A, No. 5 (Jan. 1979), p. 136.

CHAPTER 8   HOW THE PILL CAN SPOIL SEX

"Pill gets no credit for rise in female libido, study says," *Psychiatric News* 6:9 (1971).

"Find sexual pleasure abetted in only 39% of group on pill," *Medical Tribune* (Sept. 8, 1971).

B. Seaman, *Free and Female* (Greenwich, Conn.: Fawcett, 1972).

R. P. Michael, "Hormones and sexual behavior in the female," *Hospital Practice* 10:69–76 (1976).

B. Seaman and G. Seaman, *Women and the Crisis in Sex Hormones* (New York: Bantam, 1977).

CHAPTER 9   STERILITY AND THE PILL

Royal College of General Practitioners, *Oral Contraception and Health* (1974).

S. Harlap and A. M. Davies, *The Pill and Births: the Jerusalem study. Final Report, Jan.* 1978 (Bethesda, Md.: Department of Health, Education, and Welfare, National Institute of Child Health and Development, Center for Population Research, 1978).

M. P. Vessey, N. H. Wright, K. McPherson, and P. Wiggins, "Fertility after stopping different methods of contraception," *British Medical Journal* 1(6801):265–67 (Feb. 4, 1978).

See also:

M. J. Whitelaw, V. F. Nola, and C. F. Kalman, "Irregular menses, amenorrhea and infertility following synthetic progestational agents," *Journal of the American Medical Association* 195:780–82 (1966).

J. C. Marshall, P. I. Reed, and H. Gordon, "Luteinizing hormone secretion in patients presenting with post-oral contraceptive amenorrhea," *Clinical Endocrinology* 5:131–43 (1976).

R. E. Evrand et al., "Amenorrhea following oral contraception," *American Journal of Obstetrics and Gynecology* 124:88 (1976).

D. T. Janerich et al., "Fertility patterns after discontinuation of use of oral contraceptives," *Lancet* 1:1051–53 (1976).

J. E. Tyson et al., "Neuroendocrine dysfunction in galactorrhea-amenorrhea after oral contraceptive use," *Obstetrics and Gynecology* 46:1–11 (1975).

G. G. Brooks and M. R. Butcalis, "Amenorrhea following oral contraception," *American Journal of Obstetrics and Gynecology* 124:88–91 (1976).

CHAPTER 10   GENETIC CHANGES AND THE PILL

A. L. Herbst, R. E. Scully, and S. J. Robboy, "Effects of maternal DES ingestion on the female genital tract," *Hospital Practice*, 51–57 (1975).

A. Staff, R. F. Mattingly, et al., "Clinical diagnosis of vaginal adenosis," *Obstetrics and Gynecology* 43:118–28 (1974).

M. Bibbo, "Cytologic findings in female and male offspring of DES-treated mothers," *Acta Cytologica* 19:568–72 (1975).

M. Bibbo, "Follow-up study of male and female offspring of DES-treated mothers: a preliminary report," *Journal of Reproductive Medicine* 15:15 (1975).

M. Bibbo et al., "Follow-up study of male and female offspring of DES-exposed mothers," *American Journal of Obstetrics and Gynecology* 49:1–7 (1977).

J. A. Celebre, "Management of vaginal adenosis at the hospital of the University of Pennsylvania," *Journal of Reproductive Medicine* 16:293 (1976).

"Experts discuss problems of DES-related cancer," *Journal of the American Medical Association* 234:585 (1975).

National Institutes of Health, "DES Task Force is concerned about possible risks to mothers who were exposed to DES during pregnancy," press release (Dec. 1978).

S. Harlap and A. M. Davies, *The Pill and Births: the Jerusalem study* (1978).

S. Harlap, R. Prywes, and A. M. Davies, "Birth defects and oestrogens and progesterones in pregnancy," *Lancet* 1:682–83 (1975).

O. P. Heinonen, D. Slone, R. R. Monson, E. B. Hook, and S. Shapiro, "Cardiovascular birth defects and antenatal exposure to female sex hormones," *New England Journal of Medicine* 296(2):67–70 (Jan. 13, 1977).

D. Janerich et al., "Oral contraceptives and congenital limb reduction defects," *New England Journal of Medicine* 291:697–700 (1974).

D. Janerich, at Kennedy hearings (Jan. 21, 1976).

J. J. Nora and H. A. Nora, "Birth defects and oral contraceptives," *Lancet* 1:941–42 (1973).

See also:

J. Robertson-Rintoul, "Oral contraception: potential hazards of hormone therapy during pregnancy," *Lancet* 2:1315 (1974).

J. M. Reinisch, "Effects of prenatal hormone exposure on physical and psychological development in humans and animals," in: *Hormones, Behavior and Psychopathology*, E. J. Sachar, ed. (New York: Raven, 1976).

CHAPTER 11   THE PILL AND JAUNDICE, THYROID FUNCTION, . . . ETC.

A. S. Morrison, H. Jick, and H. W. Ory, "Oral contraceptives and hepatitis: A report from the Boston Collaborative Drug Surveillance Program, Boston University Medical Center," *Lancet* 1(8022):1142–43 (May 28, 1977).

M. J. Kreek, "Cholestasis of pregnancy and during ethinyl estradiol administration in the human and the rat," in *Metabolic Effects*, Salhanick et al., eds. (1969).

A. Kappas and C. S. Song, "Sex hormones, the gastrointestinal tract and the liver: Introductory comments," in *Metabolic Effects*, Salhanick et al., eds. (1969).

B. Westerholm, "The liver and the pill," *Skandia International Symposia on Alcoholic Cirrhosis and Other Toxic Hepatopathias* (Stockholm: Nordiska Bokhandelns Forlag, 1970), pp. 251–58.

Royal College of General Practitioners, *Oral Contraceptives and Health* (1974).

Boston Collaborative Drug Surveillance Program, "Oral contraceptives and venous thromboembolic disease, surgically confirmed gallbladder disease, and breast tumors," *Lancet* 1(7817):1399–1404 (June 23, 1973).

L. J. Bennion et al., "Effects of oral contraceptives on the gallbladder bile of normal women," *New England Journal of Medicine* 294:189–92 (1976).

C. Dupont, "Herpes gestationis and the pill," *British Medical Journal* 2:699 (1968).

B. Gorden, "Herpes gestationis and the pill," *British Medical Journal* 1:15–52 (1967).

R. W. Lynch and R. J. Albrecht, "Hormonal factors in herpes gestationis," *Archives of Dermatology* 9:446–47 (1966).

D. M. Mitchell, "Herpes gestationis and the pill," *British Medical Journal* 4:1324 (1966).

W. B. Shelley, R. W. Preucell and S. S. Spoont, "Autoimmune progesterone dermatitis," *Journal of the American Medical Association* 190:35–38 (1964).

G. G. Bole et al., "Rheumatic symptoms and serological abnormalities induced by oral contraception," *Lancet* 1:323 (1969).

H. Speira and C. M. Plotz, "Rheumatic symptoms and oral contraceptives," *Lancet* 1:571–72 (1969).

See also:

G. J. Gill, "Rheumatic complaints of women using anti-ovulatory drugs," *Journal of Chronic Diseases* 21:435 (1968).

J. M. Dwyer et al., "Cell-mediated immunity in healthy women taking oral contraceptives," *Yale Journal of Biology and Medicine* 48:91–95 (1975).

E. W. Barnes et al., "Phytohaemagglutinin-induced lymphocyte transformation and circulating autoantibodies in women taking oral contraceptives," *Lancet* 1:898 (1974).

I. E. Jelinek, "Oral contraceptives and the skin," *American Family Physician* 4:68–74 (1971).

W. C. Ellerbroek, "Oral contraceptives and malignant melanoma," *Journal of the American Medical Association* 206:649–50 (1968).

G. M. El-Ashiry et al., "Effects of oral contraceptives on the gingiva," *Journal of Periodontology* 42:273–75 (1971).

A. Y. Kaufman, "An oral contraceptive as an etiologic factor in producing hyperplastic gingivitis and a neoplasm of the pregnancy tumor type," *Oral Surgery* 28:666–70 (1969).

J. Lindhe and A. Bjorn, "Influence of hormonal contraceptives on the gingiva of women," *Journal of Periodontal Research* 2:1–6 (1967).

B. D. Lynn, "The pill as an etiologic agent in hypertrophic gingivitis," *Oral Surgery* 24:333–34 (1967).

CHAPTER 12 DEPRESSION AND THE PILL

Royal College of General Practitioners, *Oral Contraceptives and Health* (1974).

M. Briggs and M. Briggs, "Vitamin C requirements and oral contraceptives," *Nature* 238:277 (1972).

M. Briggs and M. Briggs, "Vitamin C and colds," *Lancet* 1:998 (1973).

M. Briggs and M. Briggs, "Oral contraceptives and vitamin requirements," *Medical Journal of Australia* 1:407 (1975).

P. Adams, V. Wynn, and D. Rose, "Effects of pyridoxine hydrochloride (vitamin B_6) upon depression associated with oral contraception," *Lancet* 1:897 (1973).

J. Otte, "Oral contraceptives and depression," *Lancet* 2:498 (1969).

E. C. G. Grant and H. Pryse-Davis, "Effects of oral contraceptives on depressive mood changes and on endometrial monoamine oxidase and phosphatases," *British Medical Journal* 3:777–80 (1968).

J. R. McCain, at Nelson hearings.

CHAPTER 13 IRRITABILITY AND THE PILL

P. Ball, "Some apparently common problems in patients taking 'the pill,'" *Journal of the Indiana State Medical Association* (Jan. 1968).

F. J. Kane et al., "Emotional change associated with oral contraceptives in female psychiatric patients," *Comprehensive Psychiatry* 10:16–30 (1969).

F. J. Kane, "Psychosis associated with the use of oral contraceptive agents," *Southern Medical Journal* 62:190–92 (1969).

A. Nilsson and P. E. Almgren, "Psychiatric symptoms during the postpartum period as related to use of oral contraceptives," *British Medical Journal* 2:453–55 (1968).

CHAPTER 14 THE PILL AND NUTRITION

B. Seaman and G. Seaman, *Women and the Crisis in Sex Hormones* (1977).

V. Wynn, "Vitamins and contraceptive use," *Lancet* 1:561 (1975).

F. McGinty and D. P. Rose, "Influence of androgens upon tryptophan metabolism in man," *Life Sciences* 8:1193 (1969).

D. P. Rose, "Aspects of tryptophan metabolism in health and disease," *Journal of Clinical Pathology* 25:17 (1972).

D. P. Rose and I. P. Braidman, "Excretion of tryptophan metabolites as affected by pregnancy, contraceptive steroids and steroid hormones," *American Journal of Clinical Nutrition* 24:673 (1971).

A. M. Shojania, "Effect of oral contraceptives on vitamin B_{12} metabolism," *Lancet* 2:932 (1971).

A. M. Shojania and G. J. Hornady, "Oral contraceptive and folate absorption," *Journal of Laboratory and Clinical Medicine* 82:869–75 (1973).

J. E. Ryser et al., "Megaloblastic anemia due to folic acid deficiency in a young woman on oral contraceptives," *Acta Haematologica* 45:319–24 (1971).

A. S. Prasad et al., "Effect of oral contraceptive agents on nutrients: II. Vitamins," *American Journal of Clinical Nutrition* 28:385–91 (1975).

M. K. Horwitt, C. C. Harvey, C. H. Dahm, "Relationship between levels of blood lipids, vitamins C, A, and E, serum copper compounds, and urinary excretions of tryptophan metabolites in women taking oral contraceptive therapy," *American Journal of Clinical Nutrition* 28:403–12 (1975).

S. Margen and J. C. King, "Effect of oral contraceptive agents on the metabolism of some trace minerals," *American Journal of Clinical Nutrition* 28:392–402 (1975).

"The pill and changes in essential trace metals," *Medical World News* 15:32 (1974).

R. C. Theuer, "Effects of oral contraceptive agents on vitamin and mineral needs: A review," *Journal of Reproductive Medicine*, 8:13–19 (1972).

"Feminins and other vitamin-mineral supplements for women taking oral contraceptives," *Medical Letter* 15:81–82 (1973).

U. Larsson-Cohn, "Oral contraceptives and vitamins: A review," *American Journal of Obstetrics and Gynecology* 121:84–90 (1975).

A. L. Luhby et al., "Vitamin B_6 metabolism in users of oral contraceptive agents," *American Journal of Clinical Nutrition* 24:684 (1971).

W. N. Spellacy et al., "The effect of estrogens on carbohydrate metabolism," *American Journal of Obstetrics and Gynecology* 114:378–92 (1972).

W. N. Spellacy, W. C. Buhi, and S. A. Berk, "The effects of vitamin B_6 on carbohydrate metabolism in women taking steroid contraceptives," *Contraception* 6:265–73 (1972).

W. N. Spellacy, "Metabolic effects of oral contraceptives," *Clinical Obstetrics and Gynecology* 17:53–64 (1974).

P. Adams, V. Wynn, and D. Rose, "Effects of pyridoxine hydrochloride . . ." (1973).

N. Whitehead, F. Reyner, and J. Lindenbaum, "Megaloblastic changes in cervical epithelium. Association with oral contraceptive therapy and reversal with folic acid," *Journal of the American Medical Association* 226:1421 (1973).

Ten-Year Progress Report on CPR Sponsored Research, Center for Population Research, Department of Health, Education, and Welfare, Public Health Service, National Institutes of Health, 1978.

R. J. Kutsky, *Handbook of vitamins and hormones* (New York: Van Nostrand Reinhold, 1973), pp. 71–78.

J. B. Alperin, "Folate metabolism in women using oral contraceptive agents," *American Journal of Clinical Nutrition* 26:xix (1973) (abstract).

A. Paton, "Oral contraceptives and folate deficiency," *Lancet* 1:418 (1969).

A. M. Shojania, G. J. Hornady, and P. H. Barnes, "The effect of oral contraceptives on folate metabolism," *American Journal of Obstetrics and Gynecology* 111:782 (1971).

L. F. Wetalik et al., "Decreased serum B_{12} levels with oral contraceptive use," *Journal of the American Medical Association* 221:1371 (1972).

O. Martinez and D. A. Roe, "Diet and contraceptive steroids as determinants of folate status in pregnancy," *Federation Proceedings* 33:715 (1974) (abstract).

M. Briggs and M. Briggs, "Vitamin C and colds" (1973).

I. Horowitz, E. M. Fabry, and C. D. Gerson, "Bioavailability of ascorbic acid in orange juice," *Journal of the American Medical Association* 235:2624–25 (1976).

J. V. Levy and P. Bach-y-Rita, *Vitamins: Their Use and Abuse* (New York: Liveright, 1976).

R. J. Kutsky, *Handbook of Vitamins and Hormones* (New York: Van Nostrand Reinhold, 1973), pp. 71–78.

R. A. Passwater, *Super-nutrition* (New York: Pocket Books, 1976), p. 20.

C. C. Pfeiffer, *Mental and Elemental Nutrients* (New Canaan, Conn.: Keats, 1975).

I. Gal, C. Parkinson, and I. Craft, "Effects of oral contraceptives on human plasma vitamin-A levels," *British Medical Journal* 2:436–38 (1971).

CHAPTER 15   THERE ARE BETTER WAYS: ALTERNATIVES TO THE PILL

P. D. Harvey, "Condoms—a new look," *Family Planning Perspectives* 4:27–30 (1972).

J. J. Dumm, P. T. Piotrow, and I. A. Dalsimer, "The modern condom—a quality product for effective contraception," *Population Report: Barrier Methods,* Ser. H, No. 2 (1974), p. 28.

K. B. Benjamin, "Vasectomy as an office procedure," in *Foolproof Birth Control,* L. Lader, ed. (Boston: Beacon Press, 1972), pp. 82–89.

S. Kase and M. Goldfarb, "Office vasectomy—review of 500 cases," *Urology* 1:60–62 (1973).

G. Kasirsky, "After the vasectomy," in *Vasectomy, Manhood and Sex,* G. Kasirsky (New York: Springer, 1972), pp. 57–67.

Simon Population Trust, *Vasectomy: follow-up of a thousand cases* (Cambridge: Simon Population Trust, 1969).

N. N. Wig, D. Pershad, and R. P. Isaac, "A prospective study of symptom and non-symptom groups following vasectomy," *Indian Journal of Medical Research* 61:621–26 (1973).

J. Blandy, "Male Sterilization," in *Contraception Today,* A. J. Smith, ed. (London: Family Planning Association, 1971), pp. 101–7.

Margaret Pyke Center, "One thousand vasectomies," *British Medical Journal* 4:216–21 (1973).

R. E. Morgan, "Vasectomy," *Pennsylvania Medicine* 75:38–40 (1972).

J. Blandy, "Vasectomy as a method of family limitation," *Midwife and Health Visitor* 8:161–65 (1973).

H. Edey, "Psychological aspects of vasectomy," *Medical Counterpoint* 4:19–24 (1972).

K. H. Kohli and A. J. Sobrero, "Vasectomy: a study of psychosexual and general reactions," *Social Biology* 20:298–302 (1973).

R. I. Kleinman, ed., *Vasectomy* (London: International Planned Parenthood Federation, 1972).

M. D. Nickell et al., "Long-term effect of vasectomy on reproduction and liver function," *Federation Proceedings* 33:531 (1974).

S. J. Segal, "Male Fertility studies," *Contraception* 8:187–89 (1973).

E. M. Coutinho and J. F. Melo, "Successful inhibition of spermatogenesis in man without loss of libido," *Contraception* 8:119 (1973).

J. Frick, "Control of spermatogenesis in men by combined administration of progestin and androgen," *Contraception* 8:103 (1973).

H. J. Davis, *Intrauterine Devices for Contraception: the IUD* (Baltimore: Williams & Wilkins, 1971).

A. L. Southam, "Historical review of intrauterine devices," in *Intrauterine Contraception. Proceedings of the 2nd International Conference, New York, Oct. 2–3, 1964,* S. J. Segal, A. L. Southam, and D. Shaffer, eds. (Amsterdam: Excerpta Medica, 1965), pp. 3–5.

A. L. Southam, "Scale of use, safety and impact of birth control methods," *Contraception* 8:1–11 (1973).

R. P. Bernard, "Factors governing IUD performance," *American Journal of Public Health* 61:559–67 (1971).

S. C. Huber et al., "IUDs reassessed: a decade of experience," *Population Reports: Intrauterine Devices*, Ser. B, No. 2 (1975), p. 32.

United States Department of Health, Education, and Welfare, Center for Disease Control, "IUD safety: report of a nationwide physician survey," *Morbidity and Mortality Weekly Report* 23:226–31 (1974).

"Pathologist links IUDs worn for years with infertility risk," *Medical World News*, p. 50 (Apr. 14, 1980).

J. Wortman, "The diaphragm and other intravaginal barriers—a review," *Population Reports: Barrier Methods*, Ser. H, No. 4 (Jan. 1976).

M. Vessey and P. Wiggins, "Use-effectiveness of the diaphragm in a selected family planning clinic in the United Kingdom," *Contraception* 9:15–21 (1974).

Boston Women's Health Book Collective, *Our Bodies, Ourselves*, 2nd rev. ed. (New York: Simon & Schuster, 1976).

V. E. Johnson and W. H. Masters, "Intravaginal contraceptive study. Phase I. Anatomy," *Western Journal of Obstetrics and Gynecology* 70:202–7 (1962).

H. Lehfeldt, "Cervical cap," in *Manual of family planning and contraceptive practice*, M. S. Calderone (Baltimore: Williams & Wilkins, 1970), pp. 368–75.

M. Sein, "Flexible plastic contraceptive cervical caps: an ideal contraceptive for developing countries," unpublished, 1975.

CHAPTER 16   CHECK OUT YOUR CHECKUP

V. Beral, "Oral contraceptives and health," *Lancet* 1:1280 (1974).

V. Beral, "Cardiovascular disease mortality trends and oral contraceptive use in young women," *Lancet* 2:1047–51 (1976).

"Diagnostic evaluation of a woman prior to beginning contraception," *Dialogues in Oral Contraception* 1:5 (1976).

H. Jick et al., "Venous thromboembolic diseases and ABO blood type," *Lancet* 1:539–42 (1969).

Index

A Note About the Author

Barbara Seaman is the author of *Free and Female* and *Women and the Crisis in Sex Hormones,* as well as a contributor to dozens of periodicals. She has been an editor and columnist at *Ladies' Home Journal* and *Family Circle.* She is a founder of the National Women's Health Network. Educated at Oberlin, from which she holds a B.A. and L.H.D., Ms. Seaman was an advanced science writing fellow at Columbia University when she started this book. She was cited by the Library of Congress for having raised sexism in health care as a worldwide issue and also cited by the Department of Health, Education, and Welfare for introducing the concept of patient labeling on prescription drugs.

Most recently, Ms. Seaman served on the National Task Force on DES and has been a consultant to the government's Contraceptive Research Branch. She has also testified at various Senate and congressional hearings. She lives in New York City and is the mother of a son and two daughters, all "planned."

DATE DUE

APR 0 5 1994	
MAY 0 3 1994	
NOV 0 4 2004	
MAY 0 2 2006	

GAYLORD   PRINTED IN U.S.A.